PROFESSIONAL'S HANDBOOK
ON
GERIATRIC ALCOHOLISM

PROFESSIONAL'S HANDBOOK
ON
GERIATRIC ALCOHOLISM

By

DEBORAH L. SHEROUSE, C.R.C.

Licensed Mental Health Counselor
Alcohol Program Supervisor for Marion-Citrus
Mental Health Centers, Inc.
Diplomate in American Institute for Counseling
and Psychotherapy
National Association of Alcoholism Counselors

Illustrations and Graphics by

Mari O'Donnell

Mari Graphics
Ocala, Florida

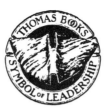

CHARLES C THOMAS • PUBLISHER

Springfield • Illinois • U.S.A.

Published and Distributed Throughout the World by

CHARLES C THOMAS • PUBLISHER
2600 South First Street
Springfield, Illinois, 62717, U.S.A.

© *1983 by* CHARLES C THOMAS • PUBLISHER

ISBN 0-398-04828-2

Library of Congress Catalog Card Number: 82-25626

With THOMAS BOOKS *careful attention is given to all details of
manufacturing and design. It is the Publisher's desire to present books that
are satisfactory as to their physical qualities and artistic possibilities and
appropriate for their particular use.* THOMAS BOOKS *will be true to those
laws of quality that assure a good name and good will.*

Printed in the United States of America

I-R-1

Library of Congress Cataloging in Publication Data

Sherouse, Deborah L.
    Professional's handbook on geriatric alcoholism.

    Bibliography: p.
    Includes index.
    1. Aged – Alcohol use. 2. Alcoholism – Treatment. 3. Aged –
Mental health services. I. Title. [DNLM: 1. Alcoholism – In old
age – Handbooks. WM 274 S552p]
RC451.4.A5S48   1983   618.97'6861   82-25626
ISBN 0-398-04828-2

To my parents,
Lollie and Barbara Sherouse,
for their example of love,
courage, and devotion.

PREFACE

THE continuing relapses of those persons over age sixty in treatment has led to the conviction that the evolving alcoholism therapy does not work as well for this population. Hence, a search for information was undertaken to explore and discern the reason for this truth.

This effort led to the realization that myths and misunderstandings about aging and about alcoholism abound not only in the general population, but in professionals as well. Most otherwise excellent treatment personnel cannot deal with the geriatric alcohol abuser.

Information regarding both fields has been sporadic and sparse. Initially, this effort was to pull together existing literature in order to learn my profession. This handbook is the extension of the concern I have for all the professional fields that encounter the elderly. Each professional is challenged to examine two basic attitudes: (1) How do I feel about growing old? and (2) What is my attitude about alcoholism?

Misdiagnosis resulting in slipshod treatment must be replaced with careful diagnosis and effective treatment. Reactive alcoholism abounds in the aged, and to treat such a person under the traditional approaches insures relapse. Thus, many of the elderly die without sobriety.

Accordingly, the handbook covers all major areas of treatment, assessment, and recovery. The ready reference format will enable the busy professional to locate and utilize information quickly. Thus, each of us can now be part of the solution to this deadly situation. My excitement abounds that this will be a reality for those I'll never meet, yet who will again become sober, useful people. To this end, I will continue to work and pray.

Debbie Sherouse
717 Southwest 16th Avenue
Ocala, Florida 32674

ACKNOWLEDGMENTS

A S always, an undertaking of this kind is accomplished with assistance from key people.

The project grew into a manuscript under the guidance of advisor, Wiley P. Mangum, Ph.D., a professor at the University of South Florida's Department of Gerontology.

The final manuscript was typed, edited and corrected by Helen Dougherty. Her secretarial expertise has made the author's job much easier.

The graphics, illustrations and much technical assistance was provided by Mari O'Donnell. Her knowledge of publications and art, plus her talent, are obvious in this work.

Special thanks must also go to my sister, Miss Linda Sherouse, for her assistance with the Bibliography and for her never-ending love and loyalty.

Thanks must also go to Mrs. Barbara Butcher for typing and to Mrs. Debbie Russell Bernard, M.S.W. for technical assistance in the aging chapters.

Perhaps the largest thanks should go to those special persons who taught me so much about alcoholism therapy. These persons are: Dr. Fred Dickman, Sandra Prince, M.S.W., Richard Poe, M.R.C., and Monica Eichberger of CompCare.

CONTENTS

PROFESSIONAL'S HANDBOOK
ON
GERIATRIC ALCOHOLISM

Chapter 1

AGING

*Aging is mind over matter; if you
don't mind, it doesn't matter.*
Satchel Paige

Aging Statistics

A NY discussion of the elderly during the decade of the 1980s has to first define who are the elderly. The 1980 United States Census count of Americans age 65 and older found that 25,544,000 Americans were in this age bracket. This is approximately 11.5 percent of the total American population in 1980. The debate has raged on for years about whether old age begins at 65 or a different age. Bernice Neugarten defines the young-old as those from 55 to 74 and the old-old as those 74 and over. This has been a defensible age breakdown for several years but is now being reconsidered by many professionals.

An American at age 65 today can expect to live another 16 years. As of 1980, the life span was 78.1 years for women and 70.5 years for men. At age 65 and older, the females outnumbered the men by a ratio of 145 to 100. During the decades of the 1980s, this life span is expected to again increase by a minimum of 3 years for both men and women.

The dilemma facing those planning future services for the elderly are multifaceted. Initially, Social Security, Supplemental Security Income, Medicare and Medicaid were intended to supplement a much smaller percentage of the elderly population. Added to the number of elderly are the number of disabled workers in younger categories who also require these benefits for their care and for the care of their family, resulting in a system that is now overburdened. This dilemma is not going to decrease based on projected figures for the future. As of the year 2000, almost 37 million Americans will be age 65 and older, or approximately 15 percent of the American population. By the year 2030, the projection is that 20 percent of the American population, or 65 million Americans, will be age 65 and older. Figure 1-1 indicates this phenomenal growth.

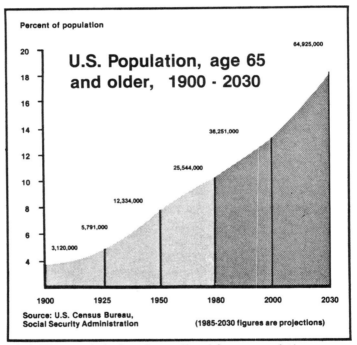

Figure 1-1. This graph depicts the predicted future population over age 65.

The White House Conference on Aging held in 1981 produced some interesting findings and recommendations. An astounding figure presented at that conference was that Americans age 55 and older totaled 45 million Americans in this country. By the year 2000, another 10 million persons will be added to that age bracket, or 55 million Americans.

To ease the Medicaid and Medicare problems being faced by the government at present, the conference recommeded for expanded federal benefits to the elderly to remain at home during serious illnesses. At present, neither Medicaid nor Medicare pays for extended home care, thus forcing the elderly person who could be managed at home to enter institutions so that their benefits can be collected. A second realization and probably the key to this whole issue is the fact that preventative medicine, including better education and health maintenance, more attention to diet, exercise and nutrition, and programs that stimulate involvement in the elderly are keys to the older American being less in need of medical care and thus less strain on the system. Both home-care funding and funding for prevention programs are two answers to the problem. For years the government has raised Social Security tax percentages and/or cut benefits instead of looking for changes that are lasting. Preventing illness is much more cost-effective than trying to fund a program to treat preventable illnesses.

Another issue facing gerontologists and the government in trying to plan for the care of the elderly is the problem of maintaining the nation's future-aged population's income. In times of a tight economy and economic stress, this is certainly no easy task. Numerous proposals are being looked into as to the feasibility of providing income for the elderly that would be adequate to maintain an acceptable level and standard of living for these Americans without increasing Social Security taxes, or other governmental taxes. In the long range, it's unknown at this point what will be done to insure that the older years for these Americans can have some stability and comfort. The tight economy is also difficult for older Americans because, while the cost of living is rising, jobs for this age group are decreasing.

In fact, unless someone is working with a company or in a program that they have been employed in for a number of years, chances are very good they cannot find a job. Certainly the post-World War II baby boom has also made this problem even more acute because of the competition of these individuals in the job market. Also, present retirement and Social Security laws that penalize workers over sixty-five after they reach a certain level of income has discouraged people from remaining in the work force because to do so would actually cost them money instead of help their standard of living improve.

Certainly the generation nearing seventy at the present time has a wealth of experience, of sacrifice, and of change on which to look back. This generation has seen the horse and buggy become sleek automobiles travelling down massive interstates, on which one can travel from one end of the country to another in a matter of days. This generation has been through four wars — two of them world wars and two of them limited conflicts — plus a world wide depression. They have seen the Wright Brother's feeble effort in an airplane become a space shuttle that flies into space and returns like an airplane to land on a runway. To quote President Ronald Reagan, "We have fought harder, paid a higher price for freedom and done more to advance the dignity of mankind than any people who have ever lived." Certainly this is an accurate assessment.

The changes in medicine and chemotherapy for various illnesses, the body of knowledge from which to draw vaccines to prevent diseases that as recently as 1950 and 1960 were killing people by the hundreds of thousands, indeed has produced a great deal to keep up with.

In spite of all this progress, this nation is ill equipped to deal with its aged populations, their needs, their concerns, and the contributions that they can still make to their country.

Research studies administered in all age groups of normal aging have produced a conviction that ignorance abounds in terms of what is normal and what lies in store for someone age sixty, seventy, or eighty in this present day. The misconception about the aging process actually has created needless worry and stress on those nearing this age bracket. Myths evolve partly because of electronic media and the press, but largely because education replaces fear and the education has not been as forthcoming as is needed. America is presently in a position of either learning what faces these people and educating them or having a crisis situation in another few years that requires a crisis solution. Certainly the research into the quality of life and how to sustain that must become both a research and a clinical priority.

Nobody suddenly wakes up one day at age 65 to discover that

they have become old. Aging is a lifelong process. Aging certainly doesn't mean that illness or a severely limited life is inevitable. And, although the National Mental Health Association has determined that approximately 25 percent of today's elderly has some degree of mental illness, this is not inevitable either. The majority of the mental health problems seen in the elderly are stress, depression, and an inability to have planned ahead and to concentrate on making the most of the life that they have ahead of them. Those who see their so-called "twilight years" as one of opportunity and new challenges certainly live a higher quality of life than those who are bogged down trying to keep circumstances as they once were.

Developmental Tasks

Many clinicians are most effective when thinking in terms of developmental tasks. The develpmental tasks that the elderly are called upon to accomplish are —

1. Adjustment to death — the "ultimate loss" (self, spouse, friends).
2. Adjustment to vocational role change (retirement — "on the shelf").
3. Adjustment to gradually failing health/physical slowdown.
4. Adjustment to reduced income.
5. Adjustment to changing living patterns (efficiency apartment, retirement community, nursing home).
6. Adjustment to the "attenuated family" (children and relatives physically removed).
7. Adjustment to changing social role ("no one listens to an old man").
8. Adjustment to physical changes in appearances.

Although these tasks are especially difficult for those who have habitually experienced failure and low self-esteem as an adult, even individuals who have coped successfully with earlier adversities and have a good self-image may experience trouble handling any of these adjustments. To compound the problems of adjustment, the older person is often faced with the loss of the very internal and external resources he had called upon previously to cope with other problems.

Several key areas need to be concentrated on in teaching the elderly what the quality of mental health in the later years can be like for them. In preparing to enter any one of these tasks in this age bracket, some general guidelines are as follows:

1. The elderly must set new goals and work towards them. This may be a new concept, but more than likely this is a concept that clients have pursued for most of their lives but have just become unable to determine what kind of goal in their older years is realistic and desirable. Often it's just a matter of deepening and clarifying some way of modifying and adapting their life long interests and attitudes toward their new situation. This problem is the most common in newly retired men and women.

2. They must learn to adapt to the changes and circumstances around them. Often a newly retired couple will decide to move to a new location to spend their retirement years in a way that they sense will be more fulfilling, but this means leaving old friends, their grown children, business acquaintances, the family home, a drop in income, perhaps even a church that they have been a major part of for a significant number of years. Such decisions need to be very carefully weighed out and discussed prior to being made. Such issues need to be thought about as what will the new area hold for them as opposed to the home and society in which they now live. What's going to happen if this move is made and one of them dies? And similar kinds of issues. This is particularly important for those on limited income who want to make the move and may not have the resources to make the move back if it's not a good decision that they have made.

3. Another major area requiring adaptation is that of retirement. The way in which the career worker retires is very significant in the process of alcohol addiction. If the worker, particularly those workers sixty years old and over, are being pressed by management to have a certain kind of output or be retired, this stress will lead to burnout and frequently cause growing dependence on alcohol. If the worker finally succumbs to such pressure, the major source of self-image is crushed making full-blown alcohol addiction possible in twelve to eighteen months. This scene is not any different during times of economic stress and high

unemployment. The combination of circumstances produces younger workers rising up and being given jobs that the older worker has been employed in for a significant number of years. Sometimes this phenomenon occurs at the expense of the most dedicated employees in a given area.

Retirement years are crucial in other major areas:

Marriage

This is often the first time since courtship that the couple has been alone together. Throughout careers and child rearing most of a couple's time is spent apart. Conversation often centers on the children, house affairs and current needs. The major thrusts in middle income families are financial security, child rearing, and establishing one's self in a profession, which is often including the career oriented wife for the last twenty years.

Sexuality

For many couples, sexuality is for procreation and either fades in importance or ceases altogether after a desired number of children are born. Most couples do not give a significant amount of thought to sexuality in the older years. Often those who have considered sexuality have been given a lot of misinformation concerning their sexuality. Certainly the myth of the dirty old man has not helped any.

Sexuality in this age group can be the most satisfying and enjoyable of any time during life. Once the woman has completed menopause, the fear of pregnancy no longer will keep the woman from enjoying her sexuality fully. For the man without business pressures and other problems that have perhaps affected him in the past, sexuality should be one of the most enjoyable experiences at this time in his life. The fact that the children are raised and that the time together can be meaningful and close should encourage couples to explore this sexuality and enjoy it as never before. The whole area of sexuality is one in which much greater emphasis must be given, and physicians, especially, need to be aware of their role as educators in this process. Elderly persons seeking to understand what is "normal" need honest, frank answers. Most elderly persons who do ask honest questions encounter embarrassment and inaccurate information.

One suprising statistic is that sexual activity does not vary between married men and unmarried men. Those who were sexually active as younger men will be sexually active in their older years.

Being married, however, greatly influences whether a woman will attempt activity. Most women who participated in one of the several studies on the subject indicated that the major deterrent was the availability of a socially acceptable sexual partner. Also, alternate methods of sexual satisfaction were usually not used.

For older persons who have received treatment for depression, education is most important. Declining sexual activity is common during depressive reactions. Many persons decide that declining sexual interest is a result of age rather than depression.

A major reason for interrupted sexual satisfaction is loss of privacy. This seems to be true for those living with their adult children as well as those who are confined to nursing homes and congregated living facilities.

One last area of sexual satisfaction comes from the increasing number of couples who marry after widowhood. No reason exists for denying those desiring to do so from enjoying the emotional, social, and sexual satisfaction. Those who remarry extend their lives. As with any couple, marriage should occur between two individuals with common values and interests. The marriage relationship is always to provide companionship and love for one another.

Avocation

A major area of adjustment is that of choosing and pursuing enjoyable activities. Much of the depression that is seen in the elderly is because of the loss of the work role, which was a major portion of the time usage during the week. Since the job is removed, finding enjoyable activities to fulfill those times is often difficult for a great many people. The surest way to overcome loneliness and isolation is to be involved with organizations. This may have already been an interest for a good number of years but for which the working person did not have the time to become involved.

For the men, this might mean coaching a Little League team, becoming involved with Boy Scouts, or any number of activities that demand an investment of time and self that otherwise possibly wouldn't be feasible for someone working. For the woman, this might be volunteerism or any number of women-oriented groups that deal with various segments of the population.

For women experiencing the "empty nest" syndrome, they can benefit by doing some volunteer work for a day agency or a foster-care agency. Involvement with grandchildren is a most rewarding opportunity for both the senior citizen and the child.

Financial

The loss of a regular paycheck and a reduced income accounts for much of the anxiety that the elderly experience. Much careful planning must be done in order to assure financial security. Many senior citizens are successful because their planning included reducing the home mortgage and paying off the automobiles. Thus the major strains are reduced to zero.

Health

Enough emphasis has not been placed on the need to pursue health insurance so that a major financial loss is not incurred should injury or illness occur. For example, a myocardial infarction can cost an individual upwards of $20,000 if not adequately covered by insurance. No one can predict when a heart problem, cancer, a fall resulting in fractures or similar dreaded catastrophes may occur. Careful exploration of available coverage from a reputable, licensed company should be investigated. The American Association for Retired Persons, Grey Panthers and similar organizations for the aged can assist with health insurance information.

Much of the adjustment of growing older is one of attitude towards our aging process. We live in an ageist society. The ageism experienced has caused people to be somewhat insecure about themselves, to overreact to aging-related difficulties, and to go to extremes in trying to be young. This has included attempting to look young, dress young and involve one's self in activities that are clearly beyond the physical capabilities of the person. However, the other extreme is just as true. This extreme includes people who retire to a rocking chair many years before they physically or mentally need to retire.

It is important for people as they grow older to realize that the stresses of aging are not avoidable in their entirety, and that a positive attitude and careful planning will help them better cope with these changes and live a more satisfying and complete life. The element of realism is vital.

Most activities in which people have been interested all of their lives can be pursued effectively during the retirement years. However, some may need to be modified. For example, a man who enjoys golfing and has formerly played eighteen holes may need to only play nine holes now on any given day. To adopt the attitude that one must complete a golf course or not play is to rob one's self of the enjoyments that one can have. Utilizing hobbies is another aspect that a great many people may have wanted to pursue, but yet, because of careers, child rearing, and possibly other limitations they have not been able to fulfill these interests either. Utilizing these strengths in the retirement years can produce one of the happiest of life-styles.

Mental changes is another area that people need to be aware of and which may include some memory loss. Minor forgetfulness is very common in all age groups. People who are concerned about forgetting important dates should write them on a calendar, which is one of the most practical and cost-effective ways of keeping track of appointments and committments. Any prolonged or pronounced memory loss needs to be investigated by a medical doctor immediately, as such is not normal aging.

The whole concept of senility has robbed people of the proper diagnosis and the proper treatment for those problems that they do have. Mental disorders in the elderly, which only affect approximately 10 percent of all persons age seventy and older, fall into two categories — organic (physical causes) and functional disorders. Organic causes include arteriosclerosis, stroke, cardiac insufficiency, and similar kinds of conditions that impair brain tissue function. There are at least ten conditions in the elderly that will cause a clinical picture of acute confusion; the first is that of alcoholism. Very few people want to deal with how large a problem this has become. If there is any reason for a physician or other treatment person to suspect that alcoholism is the problem, an assessment including a blood alcohol level should be made.

The second cause is diabetes mellitus, which is a most common condition in the elderly. The problem with diagnosing diabetes mellitus is that most doctors, if the person has never been diagnosed as diabetic before, do not look at or examine blood sugar levels to determine if this is the cause for the confusion. A blood sugar examination is a vital diagnostic tool in treating elderly, confused patients.

Thirdly, one-third of all cases of acute confusion are due to cerebral causes. These include cerebral infarctions, embolism and thrombosis. The simple absence of neurological deficiencies does not mean that a person has *not* suffered a stroke. In cases which seem not to respond or be caused by any other known or assessable cause, a cerebral spinal fluid tap will show an excess of protein if a cerebral infarction has occurred.

Fourthly, approximately half of all cases of acute confusion in the elderly are due to extra-cerebral causes. The most common causes are cardiac failure, lung disease, anemia and kidney failure. Also, a mild myocardial infarction in an elderly patient may present itself painlessly as acute confusion. When mental changes coincide with falling blood pressure, an electrocardiograph is essential to determine if the heart is in fact causing the confused state (Chartan, 1976). Also, enzyme studies can confirm if this is the cause of the person's problem.

Fifthly, any major vitamin deficit in the elderly can present itself as acute confusion. A particular liability is the B-12 deficit in elderly persons. As economic stresses and hard times continue to lower the buying power of the elderly person's limited income, nutritional deficits are going to be on the increase. These must be equally examined as the causation of acute confusion.

Sixth, acute confusion following anesthesia for major/minor surgery is very common. Hospital personnel must be reminded that anesthesia is a major chemical to introduce into a body of an older person. Because of the aging process, the body detoxifies itself from anesthesia somewhat more slowly; thus confusion is not uncommon for several days following surgery and may recur at a later time, particularly if Pentathol® was the anesthetizing agent.

Seventh, eye operations are a major cause of confusion in the elderly, and the confusion may last as long as six to nine months, depending on the type of surgery and the amount of time that the person requires to regain sight. For persons with myocular degeneration or some similar cause of blindness in the aged, confusion presents itself in a very acute form. For these individuals, referral to a blind school is highly appropriate for training and support so that independence, which is so highly valued, can be maintained.

Eighth, another key, natural change is the blunting of the thirst reflex. Elderly persons must be encouraged to drink at least a quart of water a day. Most people rarely drink plain water and only when quite thirsty and nothing else is available. For an elderly person to engage in this would cause a disturbance of salt and water metabolism, thereby creating an electrolyte imbalance that will present itself as acute confusion. Medical histories must concentrate on educating persons to drink plain water and emphasize the importance of this to their health.

Another key cause of dehydration in the elderly is the use of prescription drugs that are not sufficiently washed out of the bloodstream through adequate fluid intake. This is particularly true of patients on diuretics. Numerous elderly patients have decided that because fluid retention is a problem, to take a diuretic and cut their fluid intake will help their problems out. This approach will guarantee dehydration.

Ninth, fecal impaction is a cause of confusion in some elderly persons. This can be readily determined by a nurse performing a rectal examination, but, more importantly, assessment needs to be made as to what kind of home remedy, if any, this person may have used before coming in for medical help. It is quite dangerous to initiate certain forms of treatment if the person has been treating themselves with over-the-counter medication. Assessment must include this.

Tenth, significant depression in the elderly can often present itself as a confused state. Usually at the core of such depressive reactions is either the death of an important person of some other age or a definable loss that occurred in the individual's life. The issue is not whether the therapist views this as a major, devastating loss, but rather how the person views it. For this individual, supportive counseling and education should be utilized prior to using any medication.

Eleventh, medication overdosage is a major cause of acute confusion in the elderly. This is particularly true for those persons who have significant chronic illness and are required to take medications for two or more of these illnesses. Such medications may include digitalis, some anti-depressants, anti-parkinsonism drugs, hypotensive agents and diuretics. A careful drug-taking history must be made prior to treating· any patient with any form of chemotherapy. Often an elderly person with a chronic disease can be maintained on almost half of the medications that they are currently taking at the time the confused state occurs. Again, it is significant that the organs that process and take these drugs out of the person's body slow down with older age. Thus, the person usually requires less medication but also requires more time to process the medication.

The second overall class of mental disorders are that of functional disorders. Functional disorders include many of the thought and mood disorders, loss of motivation, loss of outside interest, and acute depression. Another major cause of confusion in the elderly is sensory deprivation. If the person lives in the same environment day after day, hearing the same sounds, doing the same activity, eating the same foods and watching the same television shows, eventually the person can function only in that environment. If the person for any reason is moved to another environment, an acutely confused state will present itself. For these individuals, orientation, simple assistance and adjustment are quite important, and often the indivdual requires no more than this.

If the person has a lifetime of previous psychiatric difficulties, then a mental health clinic may be a preferable place to seek assistance. Some functional disorders can also present themselves in the environment and need only some reorientation and rearranging of the environment to deal with them. For example, someone who has trouble taking medication on time or remembering if they have taken their medication can simply label the slots in an egg carton with the the times and the medication in the appropriate slots for that day. Thus, if they have problems remembering whether or not they have taken it, they simply look in the egg carton, and if it is there they have not taken it and if it is gone they have taken it.

Also, motivational loss can often be traced to a negative attitude toward aging or to a major move in which new friends have not been made and their activities have not been rewarding. Such difficulties are treated quite effectively through the use of a volunteer program or through the use of short-term psychotherapy. By utilizing volunteers, the person can be introduced to the community and involved in various activities. This approach is particularly successful when transportation has been an obstacle.

Mental Health Issues

Unquestionably, the elderly are asked to deal with losses in varying degrees and with varying responses.

The concept of cumulative loss is not new when applied to the elderly. The list of losses with which they must deal is presented in the Cumulative Loss Pyramid (see Fig. 1–2). The therapeutic intervention requirements are also presented in the pyramid.

While the therapist issues and therapeutic techniques are discussed in detail in Chapter 6, "Mental Health/Psychotherapy," a few pointers are worth examination.

First, all people have a so-called "breaking point." Many have expressed during treatment, "I never expected this to get to me." When such "breaks" are dealt with ahead of time, then the occurrence might well be less devastating.

The continued rise in suicides among the elderly within the first six months following the death of the spouse highlights this point. Despite the improbability that both spouses will die at the same time, the surviving spouse is finding it increasingly difficult to remain alive.

Secondly, personal values influence how someone will adjust to personal losses. For example, deep religious convictions often help with the grief experienced following deaths of significant persons. Many religions teach against materialism and dependence

CUMULATIVE LOSS PYRAMID°

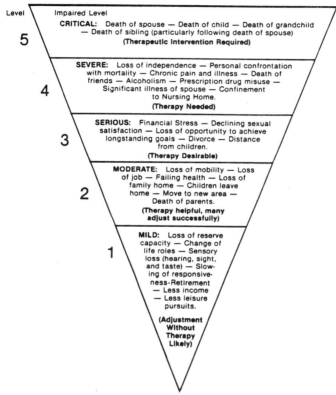

Level

Impaired Level

CRITICAL: Death of spouse — Death of child — Death of grandchild — Death of sibling (particularly following death of spouse)
(Therapeutic Intervention Required)

5

SEVERE: Loss of independence — Personal confrontation with mortality — Chronic pain and illness — Death of friends — Alcoholism — Prescription drug misuse — Significant illness of spouse — Confinement to Nursing Home.
(Therapy Needed)

4

SERIOUS: Financial Stress — Declining sexual satisfaction — Loss of opportunity to achieve longstanding goals — Divorce — Distance from children.
(Therapy Desirable)

3

MODERATE: Loss of mobility — Loss of job — Failing health — Loss of family home — Children leave home — Move to new area — Death of parents.
(Therapy helpful, many adjust successfully)

2

MILD: Loss of reserve capacity — Change of life roles — Sensory loss (hearing, sight, and taste) — Slowing of responsiveness-Retirement — Less income — Less leisure pursuits.

(Adjustment Without Therapy Likely)

1

Figure 1-2. The pyramid categorizes types of loss experienced by the elderly and the usual severity of the loss.

on possessions for happiness, thus enabling believers to deal with loss of possessions.

Thirdly, remaining social service networks enable the person to survive major loss. Persons who remain in the same locality and are involved in the community throughout the years can usually count on abundant assistance during times of loss and stress.

Psychological Changes

The following are the changes that occur in most people to some degree in late life.

I. Personality Traits
    A. Tendency toward rigidity
    B. Greater tolerance for ambiguity
    C. Increase in cautiousness
    D. Increase in self-concern
II. Intelligence, Learning and Memory
    A. Intelligence
        1. Fluid intelligence — innateability or physiological potential to deal with intellectual materials. Tends to increase into early adulthood and then decline.
        2. Crystallized intelligence — based on cultural learning. Tends to increase gradually throughout adulthood.
    B. Learning
        1. Decrements in performance on learning tasks with age
            a. Input–output problems
            b. Loss of speed
            c. Motivational elements
            d. Health status
            e. Fear of failure
            f. Anxiety
    C. Memory
        1. Short-term recall deficits
        2. Long-term memory remains intact
        3. Greater time required for memory scanning
    D. Life review process
        1. Depressive reactions to goals not accomplished

Suicide

The suicide rate in 1980 in America for persons over 65 was 22.9 per 100,000. In retiree areas, such as Miami Beach, Florida, the rate increases 38 percent to 31.7 per 100,000. However, for those over age 75 the Miami Beach rate skyrockets to 61.2 per 100,000, or 180 percent higher than the national average.

Similar other areas report similar findings. The at-risk populations are poor, Caucasian, of frail health and those experiencing major loss of another in their life.

Foster Grandparents

Foster grandparents is a super program for those elderly person's who have the time, are motivated and in good health so they can provide a child a grandparent who loves them and does all the things that grandparents are noted for doing when they love a child. Perhaps, however, for the lonely, isolated elderly, this is exactly backwards. Perhaps there should be a program to adopt a grandparent, whereby people in their teens, twenties and thirties actually adopt the elderly to be their grandparents and spend time loving them like a young adult can love back a grandparent. This would also eliminate a lot of the loneliness and failure to have needs met that many of the isolated elderly have experienced.

Could we imagine being in our twenties and having no one in the world who is a blood relative? Could we imagine not having parents, a brother, sister, an aunt or uncle, a spouse, a child that is our relative whom we can love and who loves us back? And yet this is precisely the kind of situation in which many elderly are finding themselves as they outlive everybody in their family system, no matter how remote a relative. This sets the person up for loneliness, for depression, for alcoholism and for any numerous other kinds of things to happen to a person who has no one else.

Death Issues

There is an incredible myth in this society that any discussion of death hastens its approach. Therefore, death is denied, feared and misunderstood because of the superstition that talking about death means one will die sooner. For the senior citizen, this is a double bind. They are closer to death (as far as natural causes) than their younger counterparts in society. The double binding, because of the superstition, prevents planning for death, arranging for a funeral, or even making out a will, because this planning is seen as morbid and unnatural. Of course, the only time this is really true is for the suicidal person who is making the final arrangements because they have planned to take their lives in the near future. While the expectation for a great many years of life ahead of us is less for someone in their sixties or seventies than it is for someone in their twenties or thirties, the fear that these people have of impending death can be seen, rather than fatalistic, as being an ingredient of reality.

The therapeutic approach to someone unduly concerned and preoccupied with their life running out is to help them plan what would be meaningful for them at this time in their lives and help them implement a plan of participating in those activities, seeing those people and enjoying the areas of their lives that mean the most to them. The fear of nearing death certainly places illnesses, which would not be traumatic for a forty or fifty-year-old, in a whole different light for a seventy or eighty-year-old. An illness that takes three to five months recovery is a more devastating blow to someone in the old-old category, because three to five months may be a major portion of the time that they have left in their lives. When such an individual who has an illness presents themselves for support, they need to be given this. To the individual who is in their seventies or eighties, they may think, "How many more periods of three to five months might I have left in my life." Thus, the illness is viewed as robbing them of their last remaining chances to do a good many things in which they may wish to be involved. This is particularly true for approximately 90 percent of all elderly persons in this country. Those who have no major restrictions on their mobility or their health and have been able to engage in different activities may have found this rewarding and useful in their twilight years. Such an illness is now indeed more than they know how to cope with or bear.

This whole idea of not being able to discuss death and fears about death must be dealt with openly in a factual, calm, therapeutic manner with such individuals. The more information that is given and available concerning death — the life-after-death issues, religious issues and issues of how and why the body might shut itself down — then the easier it is for someone to face that impending possibility. Some persons will never even consider death or think about impending death until a serious illness in their retirement years. At that point, the thoughts and feelings concerning death may very well be of an hysterical nature and need gentle, factual dealing from a person who is comfortable discussing death and all the componenets of the dying process with such an individual.

The Death Attitude Questionnaire helps facilitate discussions of these issues in an open, supportive manner (see Fig. 1-3).

DEATH ATTITUDE QUESTIONNAIRE

1) I believe life is:
2) I believe death is:
3) When I think about my death I:
4) If I could choose my way to die (not suicide), I hope it is:
5) Religious belief influences my feelings about death because:
6) The Religious belief I hold helps most with:
7) If I planned my own funeral I would want:
8) When I die, I'd like to be buried/or cremated because:
9) If one member of my family died, I would feel:
10) When my patients die I feel:
11) My feelings regarding suicide are:
12) If _____ happened, I might feel as though suicide was a viable option.
13) A beautiful death process is:
14) I want to die before my spouse or I want my spouse to die first because:
15) The ideal age for me to die is:

Figure 1-3. Attitudes about death often need to be explored. This tool gives therapists a constructive framework in which to discuss death. This is most useful to those therapists who are unsure of how to counsel the terminal or grieving client.

The movement of hospice in this country as a carry-over from England has been particularly effective in doing this for cancer victims and their families. Certainly the possibility of dying looks squarely in the eyes of a cancer victim and, of course, is something that must be dealt with within their family unit. What hospice has done, meaningfully so, is provide counseling and education, support and comfort for the victims and for their families at a time when most need such services. This has made the dying trajectory for the patients much more comfortable and has enabled the family to adjust and deal with the grief process in the most effective way yet discovered. What needs to be done as a natural outgrowth of hospice is for such information to be available to all elderly people to help them deal with the fears and concerns as they arise that they have about dying.

For some elderly individuals, death is first experienced through the death of a spouse, a child or grandchild, or a close friend. Some of these individuals may never have been involved in the death of someone close to them. In fact, many young–old (54–70 years) in today's society still have parents living.

Physical Changes After Age Fifty-five

The physical changes that occur for all persons over the later part of life are presented in outline form for easy professional reference.

Skin (Integument)

1. Wrinkling due to loss of skin elasticity and decreased subcutaneous fat.
2. Graying and loss of hair.
3. Appearance of brown pigmented spots on back of hands, wrists, and face.
4. Small hemorrhages under the skin due to thinness of skin and increasing fragility of small blood vessels.
5. Increased toughness and brittleness of fingernails and toenails.
6. Skin becomes very dry.

Musculoskeletal System

1. Atrophy of muscles.
2. Loss of muscle elasticity.
3. Loss of bone mass; bones become more porous or less dense (osteoporosis).
4. Back pain due to age-related changes in vertebral discs of spinal column.
5. Postural changes
6. Changes in mobility due to decreased body flexibility.

Nervous System

1. Changes in nerve cells.
   a. Loss of neurons.
   b. Increase in supporting tissues of brain and spinal cord.
2. Appearance of a brownish pigment (lipofusin) in nerve cells.
3. Lessening of biochemical activity.
4. Blood circulation to cerebral area is reduced; less oxygen utilized.

5. Changes in transmission efficiency.
6. Changes in brain-wave patterns.
7. Changes in sleep patterns.
8. Changes in autonomic nervous system.
   a. Slowness of functioning.
   b. Prolonged recovery time needed after activation.

Sensory Systems

1. Vision.
   a. Increase in visual threshold (i..e. more light needed).
   b. Decrease in visual acuity.
   c. Decrease in pupil size.
   d. Changes in the lens.
2. Hearing (audition).
   a. Presbycusis — loss of high-frequency sounds.
   b. Changes in ear membranes, which become thickened and more rigid.
   c. Thickening of ear wax (cerumen).
3. Taste (gustation).
   a. Decline in number of taste buds.
   b. Heightened threshold of remaining taste buds.
4. Smell (olfaction).
   a. Decline in number of fibers in the olfactory nerve.
5. Skin senses (cutaneous).
   a. Loss of receptors and increased threshold of stimulation.
6. Vestibular and kinesthetic senses.
   a. Higher thresholds of stimulation and decreased behavioral efficiency.
   b. Impairment of equilibrium and balance when fast movement is required.

Circulatory System

1. Structural changes.
   a. Increase in amount of fatty tissue in the heart.
   b. Thickening and rigidity of heart valves.
   c. Thickening, hardening and lessened elasticity of blood vessel walls (especially in arteries).
2. Functional changes.
   a. Older heart muscle requires a longer time to recover after each beat.

    b.   Heart arrhythmia more common.

    c.   Decline in cardiac output, thus providing less oxygen to body tissues and organs.

Respiratory System

1. Skeletal changes (calcification of rib cartilage, osteoporosis, kyphosis, scoliosis) limited rib cage expansion.
2. Weakening and atrophy of muscles responsible for inhalation and exhalation.
3. Lungs become less elastic, thus reducing vital capacity.
4. Decrease in number of capillaries surrounding the alveoli and an increase in the thickness of the alveola and capillary membranes.

Digestive System

1. Changes in the mouth.
   a. Decrease in the number of taste buds on the tongue.
   b. Decrease in secretion of salivary and digestive glands.
   c. Increase in the thickness of mucin.
   d. More alkaline saliva.
   e. Some shrinking of bony structures.
2. Changes in the esophagus.
   a. Decrease in peristalsis.
   b. Delay in emptying contents due to less frequent openings of sphincter muscle in lower esophagus.
3. Changes in the stomach.
   a. Reduced gastric mobility due to loss of muscle tone.
   b. Reduction in stomach volume.
   c. Shrinkage of mucous membranes in the stomach.
   d. Decline in the number of gastric cells.
   e. Reduction in secretion of both hydrochloric acid and enzymes.
4. Changes in the intestines.
   a. Decreased tone of intestinal muscle.
   b. Loss of elasticity of abdominal muscles.
   c. Shrinkage of the mucous lining and a decline in number of absorbing cells.

Urinary System

1. Decrease in nephrons.
2. Decrease in renal blood flow.

3. Declining bladder capacity.

Reproductive System

1. Female System.
   a. Climacteric marks the end of menstruation and coincides with the cessation of reproductive ability and decreased amounts of estrogen and progesterone are produced by the ovaries.
   b. External genitalia shrink somewhat and there is a decrease of pubic hair.
   c. Vaginal canal becomes pale, dry, thin and less elastic. Glandular secretions in the cana decrease and PH is less acidic.
   d. Ovaries and uterus decrease in size and the uterus becomes more fibrous.
   e. Ligaments supporting these structures tend to lose elasticity.
   f. Muscle and glandular tone diminish and skin is less elastic resulting in loss of firmness of breast and other body tissue.
2. Male System.
   a. Male climacteric usually occurs between the ages of 48 and 60.
   b. Testosterone levels decline, resulting in a decrease in size and firmness of the testes and more dense seminiferous tubules.
   c. Fewer sperm are produced and sexual energy lessens somewhat.
   d. Amount and consistency of seminal fluid changes and ejaculatory force is diminished.
   e. Increase in size of prostate gland.
   f. Sexual excitement during stimulation develops more slowly as does erection, although erection can be sustained for a longer period of time before ejaculation occurs.

Endocrine System

1. Gradual reduction in hormal secretions of the adrenal glands and the gonads.

Summary Statements

1. Chronological age is not a reliable predictory of specific organ system efficiency or behavior.

2. In spite of individual variations, there is some loss of reserve capacity in all organ systems of the body with age. Stress results in reduced efficiency or inability to cope.

3. Proper nutrition, exercise, pacing and regulating the environment to the maximally supportive are positive methods of offsetting the impact of physical aging in the body systems.

4. A characteristic behavior of older age is slowness. Slowness in receiving information, slowness in processing information and slowness in reacting to information.

5. Age-related physical changes increase the possibility of accidents and injury.

6. Old age is not to be equated with illness, although the older person is more susceptible to illness.

Chapter 2

GENERAL ALCOHOL INFORMATION

Background

ALCOHOL consumption has become a problem for any individual when the negative effects of drinking are evident in the person's well-being and the well-being of others. This is true for those who are diagnosed alcoholic and their families, but it is just as true for a social drinker who becomes entangled with the law for any of a number of reasons.

The extent of the problem is awesome. A recent *Harvard Medical Letter* stated the count of alcohol-addicted persons in the United States is twenty million. Additionally, every alcoholic affects a minimum of four persons in the illness process. Statistically, this means twenty million addicted persons, plus eighty million significant others, which totals ONE-HALF THE AMERICAN POPULATION in need of treatment for alcohol-related illness!

Added to this already bleak picture is the fact that there are very few pure alcoholics. In fact, recent research indicates as many as two-thirds of all the persons seeking alcoholism treatment are cross-addicted to a minimum of one other substance. Dodie Gust deals with this subject in her pamphlet, *Up, Down and Sideways on Wet and Dry Booze.* *

> In 1974 during a week-long conference in which the medical authorities on alcoholism met to discuss the disease, an informal discussion centered on the growing use of other drugs in combination

*From Dodie Gust, *Up, Down and Sideways on Wet and Dry Booze,* 1977. Courtesy of CompCare Publications, 2415 Annapolis Lane, Minneapolis, Minnesota 55441.

with alcohol. One of the attendants from the Lake Community asked Doctor Franka A. Seixas, Medical Director for the National Council on Alcoholism, "Do you think there is such a thing anymore as a pure alcoholic?" Seixas, "Anybody who drinks that much can't remain pure." But, humor aside, Seixas' observation contains more than a modicum of truth.

A research report released in 1976 by Comprehensive Care Corporation, a health management company which provides alcoholic rehabilitation programs in general hospitals (care units), strongly supports Seixas' statement. The research was carried out in the care unit programs in hospitals in California, Oregon, Washington and Colorado and was based on the intake sample of more than 500 patients. According to Richard A. Santoni, Ph.D., Director of Professional Services from CompCare, nearly two-thirds of the tested group stated they had used specific psychotropic drugs in addition to alcohol. The reports said 72 percent of the patients treated were male, and 28 percent were female.

Licit and illicit drugs, commenting on the one drug leads to another syndrome, Doctor Jerome H. Jaffe is quoted as saying, "such agents seem to serve the function of alerting the individual to the fact that substances exist which may be able to alter the feelings of inner tension."

Many studies in case histories substantiate this: drinking frequently leads to pill popping, and the use of "dry drugs" often leads to the use of the liquid drug, alcohol — the nation's number one drug of abuse, which has left ten million alcoholics in its wake. In the Spring, 1977 issue of *Addiction,* published by the Addictions Research Foundation of Ontario, in the article "Liberated Drinking — New Hazard for Women," authors Pulse, Whitehead and Revero consider the possibility that widespread use of pills by women is the major fact in their increase use of alcohol. They write, "A final consideration concerns a general increase in the use of all drugs in our society. During the past few decades, unprecedented increases in the uses of licit and illicit drugs have occurred. To some extent, this has been a function of the increased availability of drugs. Psychoactive drugs have been promoted and prescribed for a sizeable portion of the adult population, and women have consumed the majority of them. There is evidence that the use of any one drug is associated with an increased likelihood of the use of other drugs, including alcohol."

In 1964, 149 million prescriptions for psychotherapeutic drugs were filled in American drugstores. During the next six years, such prescriptions increased by about 7 percent a year to a total of 214 million in 1970. In 1972, there were 260 million such prescriptions filled, with anti-anxiety drugs accounting for the great bulk of the

increase. In 1973, there were 57 million prescriptions for Valium®
alone.

The latest available statistics show that more than two-thirds of
all users of psychoactive prescription drugs are women.

But this doesn't tell the whole story. Use of the psychic modi-
fiers by men is also on the upswing. Thet just get them through
other channels, preferring to obtain them informally on the gray
market from friends, girl friends, wives, or fellow drinkers in the
local watering spa. And, for people under thirty, male and female,
the gray market connection is the rule rather than the exception.

Added to this is the upswing in the number of significant
others seeking treatment for themselves who are given major and
minor tranquilizers to cope with the stress at home, which places
still another chemical in the already chemically troubled family
system. The significant other often despises the alcoholic for dealing with life on the basis of his or her drinking, but yet must deal
with the alcoholic on the basis of a bottle of tranquilizers. The
circle is vicious, painful and never ending in too many cases.

Perhaps the greatest challenge to any treatment staff is to
break into this cycle of addiction and misery and get some member of the family system successfully into treatment.

Alcohol may have become a problem for an individual when
any of the following apply:

1. They need a drink to cope with day-to-day life events. "Crisis" drinking is the rule.
2. They drink to a state of intoxication on a regular basis. For
   some this is a daily, for some this is a weekend, and for
   others it is a binge.
3. They go to work intoxicated or after drinking, or drink at
   work.
4. They drive a car after drinking two drinks in an hour's span.
5. They sustain a bodily injury as a result of being intoxicated.
   The staggering drunk is not funny — only sick.
6. They commit a criminal act of any nature while intoxicated.
   A good diagnostic question to ask such an individual is,
   Would you have committed this act had you not been drinking? If the answer is no, then the person has a drinking
   problem.
7. They injure another human being while intoxicated,

whether that injury is by fighting, car accident or abuse.

8. They suffer economic loss as a direct result of drinking. This category includes loss of job, spending rent money or other household money on drinking, or drinking to the exclusion of family well-being.

9. They continue to drink despite warnings from a physician that to do so would injure vital body organs or endanger the person's life.

10. They place the importance of drinking ahead of God, family and self.

So the valid question becomes, What causes a social drinker to escalate into alcoholism? No one cause for alcoholism has been established. Alcoholism is a complex interaction of biological, psychological and sociological factors. Researchers are examining such causes of alcoholism as genetic linkage to previous persons (i.e. within the last two generations), chemical abnormalities in the person's ability to deal with alcohol once ingested, poor nutrition, emotional problems, childhood deprivation and environmental conditions.

Alcohol does not cause alcoholism any more than marriage causes divorce. Certainly alcoholism would be impossible without alcohol; however, the simple solution of removing alcohol and thereby ending alcohol problems forever was called Prohibition. This did not work and will not work as the solution.

Prevention of the alcohol problems detailed above rests in education and early diagnosis. Alcoholism is the most treatable of the major causes of death in the world. Yet, like cancer, hypertension and heart difficulties, if alcoholism is not diagnosed and treated, the end result is death. In Chapter 15, the mortality rates ascribed to alcohol and the excess mortality issue will be discussed in detail.

Ethyl alcohol is a chemical found in beer, wine and distilled beverages. A record of alcohol-containing beverages dates back to the earliest beginning of history. Ethyl alcohol is produced by fermenting sugar in some form and yeast. Various alcoholic beverages are produced by fermenting sugar from different sources. For instance, beer is made from germinated barley. Wines are made from grapes and berries. Whiskey is produced from multi-grains, and rum is produced from molasses.

Distilled beverages are hard liquors that are further distilled so that concentrations of alcohol are further increased. This class of beverages includes scotch, gin, vodka, brandy, and some of the whiskey family. A prevalent and popular myth is that one cannot become an alcoholic if the person drinks only beer.

The Alcoholic Equivalency Chart indicates that this is not the case (See Fig. 2-1). Twelve ounces of beer, 5.5 ounces of regular wine, 3.5 ounces of fortified wine, 2.5 ounce highball or mixed drink, and 1 ounce of hard liquor contain the same amount of ethyl alcohol and will act on the person's body in the same way. The amount of alcohol in a bottle is known as proof and may be determined by dividing the proof by two (see Fig. 2-2).

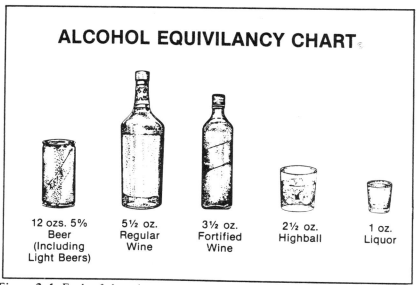

Figure 2-1. Each of these beverages contain the same amount of ethanol.

Process of Alcohol in the Body

In the Liver:

When alcohol is ingested, the liver secretes an enzyme called alcohol dehydrogenase with nicotinamide adenine dinucleotide.

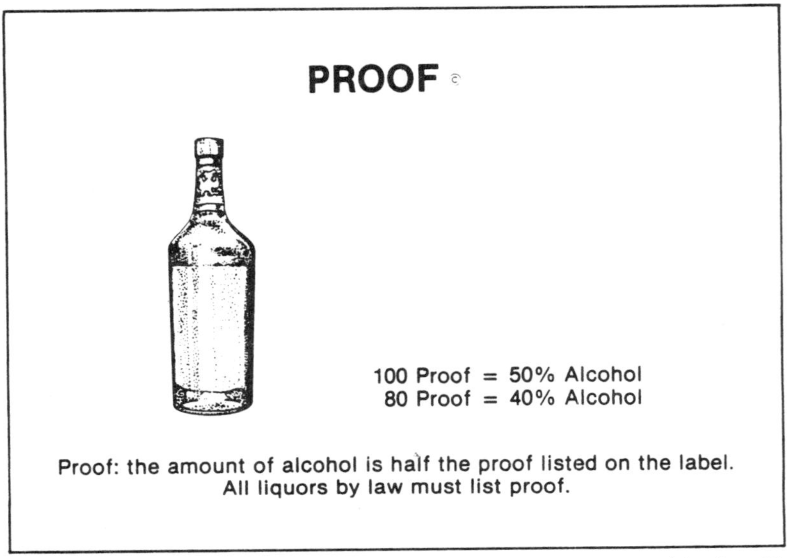

PROOF ©

100 Proof = 50% Alcohol
80 Proof = 40% Alcohol

Proof: the amount of alcohol is half the proof listed on the label.
All liquors by law must list proof.

Figure 2-2. Proof is a system for classifying certain beverages and is thus illustrated.

This starts the metabolic process. Acetaldehyde is the result of the first step in this process and it is broken down by aldehyde dehydrogenase into acetic and finally into carbon dioxide and water.

Though the metabolic steps are the same for both the alcoholic and the non-alcoholic, the resulting levels are different and higher levels of acetaldehyde are produced in the body of the alcoholic. The liver has two pathways for metabolizing ethanol. The first is known as the cytosol and the second is known as the microsomal ethanol oxydizing system (MEOS).

The cytosol is used by most people when small amounts of alcohol are ingested and it produces low amounts of acetaldehyde. The MEOS is used for metabolizing larger amounts of alcohol and it produces larger quantities of acetaldehyde. Because of an adaptational process, the MEOS becomes the primary pathway for the alcoholic and it is used to metabolize even small amounts of alcohol.

METABOLISM OF ALCOHOL

Ethanol . . . ADH- - - -Acetaldehyde . . . Aldehyde . . Acetic . . H_2O
        NAD   Dehydrogenase   Acid CO_2

Other Alcohol Excretions:

Hoffman, in his book, explains the unchanged urine and ex-pired air excretion of alcohol from the body, which accounts for 10 percent of the ingested alcohol. Primarily, this is excreted through the lungs, which validates the breathalizer test, and in the urine, which validates the urinalysis method of determining blood alcohol concentrations in a short period of time. The caution that Hoffman gives is worth considering.

The concentration of alcohol in urine is about 1.25 times greater than that in blood. The concentration of alcohol in saliva is 1.12 times greater than in alveolar air. Similarly, the concentration of alcohol in blood is 2100 times greater than in alveolar air.

Blood Alcohol Concentrations

The study of blood alcohol concentrations is one that has been debated probably far more than it needed to be in the field of treatment. Figure 2-3 indicates the possible blood alcohol concentrations for one, two and three drinks per body weight of an individual from the various classifications previously discussed. Generally speaking, any two drinks that contain the same amount of ethyl alcohol will have a similar effect on the same drinker.

Estimated Possible Blood-Alcohol Concentration Achieved With Normal Serving*

Alcoholic Beverages	Normal Servings	ONE DRINK		TWO DRINKS		THREE DRINKS	
		Alcohol Content	Body Weight 100 140 180 220	Alcohol Content	Body Weight 100 140 180 220	Alcohol Content	Body Weight 100 140 180 220
		(oz.)	(Per Cent)*	(oz.)	(Per Cent)*	(oz.)	(Per Cent)*
Beer	12 oz.	.48	.04 .03 .02 .02	.96	.07 .05 .04 .03	1.44	.10 .08 .06 .05
Wine	3 oz.	.36	.03 .03 .02 .02	.72	.06 .05 .04 .03	1.08	.08 .06 .04 .04
Liqueur	1 oz.	.40	.03 .03 .02 .02	.80	.07 .05 .04 .03	1.20	.03 .06 .05 .05
Distilled Spirits	1 oz.	.45	.04 .03 .02 .02	.90	.07 .05 .04 .03	1.35	.09 .07 .06 .05
Mixed Drinks							
Martini, Manhattan	3.5 oz.	1.05	.08 .06 .04 .04	2.10	.15 .12 .10 .09	3.15	.22 .16 .12 .10
Old Fashioned, Daquiri, Alexander, Margarita	4 oz.	.60	.05 .04 .03 .02	1.20	.08 .06 .05 .05	1.80	.11 .09 .08 .07
Highballs w/Mixes	8 oz.	.56	.05 .04 .03 .02	1.21	.08 .06 .05 .04	1.68	.12 .09 .07 .06

Chart Courtesy National Safety Council   This Table is Only for Educational Purposes

Figure 2-3. Blood alcohol level (BAL) by type of drink is important for the client to understand. This figure explains BAL by major drink category.

Several factors influenced the blood alcohol level (BAL), which is also called the blood alcohol concentration and the intoxication level in various literature. These factors include:

1. *Sex of the Drinker.* Recent research suggests that women may become more intoxicated than men on the same amount of alcohol and the same form of drink even when their body weights are precisely the same. The explanation for this phenomenon is that a woman generally has less body fluid and more body fat than does a man of precisely the same weight. Since alcohol does not defuse in the body fat as rapidly as it does into the bloodstream, then the concentration of alcohol in a woman's blood will be higher even though she drinks the same amount of ethyl alcohol. Another key (unproven) factor is that many women's reactions to alcohol vary throughout their menstrual cycle. Apparently, a woman will often be more affected by alcohol right before the beginning of her menstrual period. Since alcohol may thus affect a woman more at this time, adjustment of drinking behaviors needs to be made to avoid negative reactions.

2. *Whether Food is Eaten Before or While Drinking.* Alcohol is absorbed in part through the stomach and completely by the time a drink passes partway through the small intestine (duodenum). Thus, if the stomach is empty, the alcohol defuses into the bloodstream almost immediately. If food is present, this process is much slower thus lowering the rapidity of defusion into the bloodstream and the blood alcohol level.

3. *Body Weight.* The less someone weighs, the higher the blood alcohol level on a few drinks. The more someone weighs, the lower the blood alcohol level on the same number of drinks. The rapidity of defusion also influences the hours required to metabolize a drink. Figure 2-4 gives the amount of alcohol consumed in an hour and then the approximate number of hours required to metabolize it. Important to note is that this is assuming all the body organs involved are healthy and that the person is experiencing no other health problems.

4. *Health of the Drinker.* If the person's body organs are impaired, a small amount of alcohol can have a devastating effect, particularly in the stomach (colitis, spastic colon, or

HOURS TO METABOLIZE DRINKS

Drinks*   Weight:

	100 lbs.	120 lbs.	140 lbs.	160 lbs.	200 lbs.	240 lbs.
1	3.1	2.6	2.2	1.9	1.5	1.0
2	6.2	5.2	4.5	3.9	3.0	2.0
3	9.3	7.8	6.7	5.8	4.5	3.0
4	12..4	10.4	9.0	7.8	6.0	4.0
5	15.6	13.0	11.1	9.8	7.5	5.0
6	18.6	15.6	13.5	11.7	9.0	6.0

*Drink 1½ oz. 86 proof liquor or 5 oz. 12% wine or 12 oz. 4.5% beer

*Health of all body organs is assumed in this tabulation.

Legend 2-4. The number of hours required to metabolize drinks are important to understand for the drinker who believes coffee or cold showers will enhance sobriety.

ulcer) or liver (cirrhosis or fatty liver). This is most logical, since these organs must deal with the alcohol ingested and thus incur the greatest amount of organ stress.

Should the individual suffer from allergy, asthma, cold, fever, or viral infection, a drink mixed with medication can produce toxic and sometimes fatal results. Most prescriptions are labeled, yet the warnings are frequently ignored. Anyone suffering from a chronic disease should never take a drink in any setting. These diseases include arthritis, heart disease, emphysema, asthma, kidney disease, and any form of epilepsy and diabetes. Frequently, anyone suffering from one or more of these conditions is already being treated with some form of medication. But, more importantly, these already-diseased organs cannot deal with the stress of the body excreting the alcohol.

5. *Emotional State of the Drinker.* Anyone under treatment for any form of psychiatric or mental health disorder should avoid

drinking any alcoholic beverage. Since alcohol is a central nervous system depressant, alcohol will exacerbate any functional or psychiatric disorder. Particular at-risk cases are those being treated for depression, insomnia and stress disorders. The suicide potential for these persons triples when drinking and skyrockets beyond measurements if the person is being treated with chemothrapy and then drinks. Likewise, giving a person an anti-depressant and then giving the body a generous dose of ethyl alcohol produces opposite pulls in the body at the same time. Added to this stress on the organs is that two opposite drugs must be oxidized by the liver simultaneously and the brain is both being lifted and depressed simultaneously. In an elderly person this can result in an immediate death, often classified as a natural cause. Accidental suicides also occur in these people frequently when alcohol is mixed with painkillers and/or sleeping pills. All professionals need to concentrate on educating clients to this risk. Figure 2-5 indicates areas of the brain affected by blood alcohol levels and the level required for the resulting consequences. Another significant point to remember is that dependence on alcohol often begins at the emotional or feeling level. When someone believes they need a drink to relax, to sleep, to give a speech, to facilitate communications, or for any reason instead of utilizing their inner resources, then harmful dependency on alcohol has begun. The fact is that alcohol will not enable someone to do anything while drinking that the person cannot do better sober. The process continues to include more credit given to the alcoholic beverage than the self-containing inner resources. Thus, a marriage to alcohol begins and the individual's self-worth decreases. The process can and does result in the assassination of individual self-respect and self-love. Reality is that the individual alone thinks, acts and does, not whatever the person consumes. However, this reality too can be devastating as the inevitable behavioral deterioration proceeds.

6. *Situation in Which the Person Drinks.* Drinking behavior very significantly depends on where and with whom an individual drinks. This situation must also be considered in evaluating relapses that occur. Has a person slipped into a situation for

EFFECTS OF ALCOHOL ON THE BRAIN

REQUIRED BALANCE FOR IMPAIRMENT	AREA OF BRAIN	CONSEQUENCES
.01 - .10	Frontal Lobe (Reason, Communication, Self Control)	1. Hours Self Inhibition. 2. False Confidence. 3. Impaired Judgment. 4. Dulled Attention. 5. Loss of Self-Control.
.10 - .25	Parietal Lobe (Sensory Control)	1. Dulled senses - sight, smell, feel. 2. Impaired writing ability. 3. Speech Disturbances - slurring, wrong words. 4. Loss of technical skills.
.15 - .30	Cerebellum (Coordination)	1. Loss of Equilibrium 2. Loss of Coordination
.20 - .30	Occipital Lobe (Visual Sensation)	1. Loss of Depth Perception. 2. Distorted images. 3. Double vision. 4. Loss of color recognition.
.25 - .50	Thallmus and Medulla (Respiration and Circulation Control)	1. Apathy. 2. Depression of respiration. 3. Circulation failure. 4. Subnormal temperature. 5. Stupor - Shock - Death.

(Adapted from Waterbury Manual)

Figure 2-5. The understanding of alcohol's interaction with the brain has not been understood. Thus, this chart will show this interaction. Notice the BAL overlap on various brain function.

which sufficient preparation was not made? This is a key question to examine in explaining the relapse process to the family. Relapses are going to happen in a percentage of the clinical cases, just as relapses occur in the treatment process of any chronic medical condition. Relapses is a term of choice, rather than "slipped, or fell off the wagon," if the medical model of alcoholism is utilized. The key to terminology is most important in the treatment of alcoholism in the elderly. Diabetic, cardiac patients, cancer patients and chronic lung disease patients are not told "they have fallen off the wagon." Errors in treatment or follow-through are treated as management and educational issues rather than moral issues.

A similar approach when used to treat alcoholism works rather well, facilitates the family's acceptance of the recovery process, and avoids unneeded and unwarranted setbacks in other treatment areas.

The process of alcoholism needs to always be kept in mind and is helpful as a perspective. No one develops a chronic illness over night. The illness progresses and, as the process takes hold, the body responds in certain measurable ways. This is also the case in alcoholics, and just as getting sick is a process, getting well is a process, also.

Certain attitudes and behaviors have been identified through clinical studies as being significant predictors of relapse potential. These are discussed in Chapter 9. Another point on blood alcohol levels is the increased risk of the driving accident based on the blood alcohol level. The establishment of this level has been debated in legislatures for quite awhile; however, Figure 2-6 gives the approximate increased risk and the number of hours a person should wait before they are able to drive safely. The fact that people do not wait is directly attributable to the 59 percent legally drunk drivers who cause fatal accidents in this country every year. Again, the problem with this statistic is not all of these people are alcoholics. In fact, frequently they are not alcoholics and, therefore, are not able to gauge how much they have had to drink or how much it is affecting them, and thus they are more ripe to cause an accident through ignorance than the alcoholic who knows how much they can drink and what it does to their body as they drink. Figure 2-6 shows the blood alcohol level in relationship to risk of an automobile accident and the amount of waiting time before being able to drive safely.

Several key symptoms indicate that a person has escalated from social drinking into heavy drinking into alcoholism. Figure 2-7 shows the progression and the symptoms that indicate the pro-

BAL. AS A PREDICTOR OF AUTO ACCIDENT

BAL.	INCREASE RISK OF DRIVING ACCIDENT	WAITING TIME	LEGAL DRIVING STATUS
.03	Slight	None	Sober
.06	2 times	4 hours	Sober
.09	5 times	6 hours	Borderline
.12	15 times	8 hours	Intoxicated
.15	25 times	9 hours	Intoxicated
.18	75 times	10 hours	Intoxicated
.21	200 times	12 hours	Intoxicated
.24	400 times	15 hours	Intoxicated

Figure 2-6. This is a helpful tool to educate drivers as to the risks being taken when driving after "a few drinks."

gression.* As a treatment instrument, this chart is most valuable, providing a checklist that can be completed by a person suspected of having alcohol-related problems. The promise contained in the treatment of alcoholism, particularly while diagnosed in the early stages, is recovery.

Congeners

Another important aspect of consuming a large amount of alcoholic beverage is that of congeners that are contained in those beverages. In beer, these chemicals are added to enhance flavor, to preserve and stabilize the beer during the canning and marketing process, to produce and promote foaming, and to give, to some extent, the amount of flavor that is contained in them. Some of these congeners in beer include: Arabic, which is a stabilizer; sodium hydrosulfite, which is a preservative; tannic acid, which by the way occurs in some coffee and teas and which is used to remove

---

*From C. Hegarty, *Alcoholism Today: The Progress and the Promise*, 1979. Courtesy of CompCare Publications, 2415 Annapolis Lane, Minneapolis, Minnesota 55441.

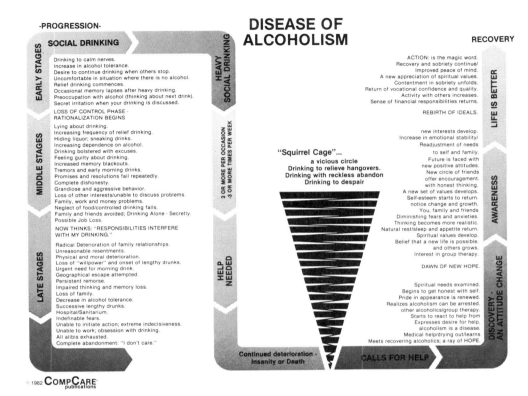

Figure 2-7. This figure first appeared in Carol Hegarty's booklet *Alcoholism Today: The Progress and the Promise* and is useful in identifying both the process of addiction and the process of recovery.

any sediment that might cause cloudiness once the beer is poured; ammonium phosphate, potassium metabisulfite, enhancers of flavor; tartaric acid, which is used to clear cloudiness; papin, although one of its properties is as a wart desolver, is added to beer to turn the beer a golden color; magnesium sulphate, otherwise known as epsom salt; amd dextrin, which is added to produce the bubbles that cause a glass of beer to foam. In other alcohols are added carbonyl compounds which is formaldehyde and acetaldehyde. These are side components or side products of the aging process of distilling some of the finer wines and brandies. Acids are also added to the distillate and are present when bottled. These are just a few of the things that are added to the many forms of ethyl alcohol on the market today. Researchers have tied many of these congeners to the cancer-causing process in the stomach, colon, lungs, liver and pancreas. It is not surprising that these things are damaging the body when consumed in increasing quantities.

Myths

The eleven most prevalent myths concerning alcohol use and abuse need to be dealt with in this chapter.

Myth 1 is that there is some other method of sobering up someone who is intoxicated besides just time. The cold reality of the situation is only time sobers up a person who is intoxicated.

Recent research indicates that giving coffee to someone and thus introducing caffeine, a stimulant, into their body may be what's responsible for some of the exaggerated staggering that some intoxicated persons do. Since it is a stimulant, it is trying to counteract the massive dose of a central nervous system depressant given the body.

Myth 2 is that if a person sticks to beer they'll never become an alcoholic. The fact of the matter is quite simple: beer contains as much ethyl alcohol as an ounce of liquor, or four ounces of wine, and will act on the body in the same way and will produce the same effect on someone who drinks it.

Myth 3 is that switching drinks will make you drunk faster or conversely help you stay sober longer than if you stick with just one alcoholic beverage. The fact is that the amount of alcohol in the drink determines how fast a person can become intoxicated, not the mixture that contains the alcohol.

Myth 4, which makes the elderly particularly susceptible to alcohol abuse, is the belief that drinking helps overcome depression. The fact is that the sedative effect may relieve anxiety for a short period of time, but these effects seldom last longer than a couple of hours. Thus, alcohol then becomes an irritant to the mind, and the person will become depressed due to the depressive action of the alcohol they have ingested.

Myth 5, which has emerged in the field within the last five or ten years, is the belief that every older drinker is a chronic alcoholic. This is not the case. Because an alcoholic dies a minimum of fifteen years sooner than their non-drinking counterpart, most alcoholics, if they are chronic, die by the age of sixty-five. The emergence of the new alcoholic or the late life alcoholic is a phenomena that treatment programs must come to grips with, especially if these people are going to be helped.

Myth 6 is the belief that few women become alcoholics. This was once true, though it is no longer the case. The ratio was once ten men for every two women who were alcoholics. The ratio is now three men to every one woman.

Myth 7 is the belief that certain races or certain religions are most apt to become alcoholics. The fact is that alcoholism is not a respector of persons, races, or socioeconomic class; it is plaguing every race, living in every area of the country, and in every age bracket. Alcoholics Anonymous has documented alcoholics as young as seven and as old as ninety-seven in their meetings.

Myth 8 which is a particularly dangerous one for teenagers is that if someone can really hold their liquor they are really doing well and are to be envied. The fact is that increasing ability to drink more and more alcohol without showing the affects of that drinking indicates increasing tolerance and is a warning sign that the alcohol-addiction process has begun. If this person continues the effects of this drinking will be devastating on them.

Myth 9 is the belief that drunkenness and alcoholism are the same thing. The fact is that many people will become drunk in their lifetime and never develop alcoholism. Many heavy drinkers that escalate into alcoholism never are drunk but drink large quantities of alcohol causing metabolic and physical change in their body that results in alcoholism.

Myth 10 is the belief that once an alcoholic recovers, the person can drink again socially. The fact is that once an alcoholic recovers, if the alcoholic truly recovers, alcohol can never again be ingested. Total abstinence for life is the only guaranteed way to prohibit a binge and a falling back into the progression to insanity and death.

Myth 11 is the belief that most alcoholics are skid row bums. The fact is that only 3 percent to 5 percent of all known alcoholics in this country are actually of the skid row or extremely chronic variety. The majority are employed, married, and able to function in a day-to-day setting but are dying of a disease that's not being treated and which will become worse without treatment.

Several outstanding treatment programs for individuals who have developed alcoholism have been developed over a period of trial and error and hard work by some very dedicated professionals. The fact that alcoholism is one of the most major killers of our American population and yet one of the most highly treatable is a double-bind tragedy. It is also a tragedy that few of us can afford to ignore much longer. The percentage is as high as 70 percent of those who enter treatment for the first time never take another drink.

The programs that treat the family also treat problems before they happen. Prevention includes bringing these families in and treating them before they develop their own serious problems. Yet, many people do not want to work with alcoholics or do not understand the process of treating an alcoholic. There are some challenges in the next section, for therapists in any human service agency, to be considered and evaluated. It is highly doubtful that anyone can remain in the human service field and not, at some point, either become overwhelmed that they cannot treat a person for alcoholism or the person will eventually have to develop an understanding of the disease and an ability to help the individuals.

Therapist Issues

Therapists can often point to the cases in which the alcoholic was obnoxious, angry, disruptive and did not quit drinking regardless of what was done by the treatment staff. The therapist must realize that not every client will succeed any more than every smoker gives up cigarettes at a smoker's clinic or every obese person forever loses weight at a weight clinic.

Yet, this issue is not simplistic. Educational level, phase of the disease, social support systems, broad-based clinical awareness of the staff, cultural pressures, religious issues, age, phase of life and marital status are all key factors in treating alcoholism.

Some clients do not achieve sobriety because the staff are not able to tailor the program to the person's needs. Black clients are often at extreme disadvantage with Caucasian staff due to lingual and racial barriers. Most programs fail to reach immigrants. Many other programs attempt to use the standard agency-approved program for all clients of all ages, races, and both sexes. These are doomed to fail a large percentage of the time.

Another key factor is the staff's attitude toward the issue of denial. Denial is *not* an attitude limited to alcoholics. Denial is a God-given reaction in each person that enables the person to have a cushion of time against the reality that is too painful to face. Each of us has reacted to a painful situation by denying the existence of the problem.

Because a stigma about alcohol addiction still exists, some clients are combative and fearful about being labeled an alcoholic. The prospect of standing up in an AA meeting and saying, "I'm _____ and I'm an alcoholic" is one which scares many people.

Mr. G was sixty-two years old. Despite obvious difficulty with alcohol, he would not deal with the concept of alcoholism. He would sit in therapy sessions and say, "I know alcohol has caused problems, but I'm not an alcoholic." The therapist then stated, "If alcohol has caused some problems, let's talk about them." Mr. G achieved sobriety, has maintained the sobriety and has made significant improvement in problems with his wife, his health and his finances.

When this client realized the term "alcoholic" was not required to achieve sobriety, he launched himself into an ambitious recovery program that was successful.

The refusal, because of fear or stigma, to be labeled an alcoholic must not keep clients from recovery. This is vital to the treatment of the elderly more than any other age bracket. Names such as "alcoholic," "drunk," and "boozer" serve to lower self-esteem and make coming into treatment much more difficult. In fact, at times it seems as though the staff has an investment in the admission of a client rather than the client.

Many hate the denial of the alcoholic and are affected by the person's denial. However, it is imperative that once the denial is broken, the self-image of the individual be rebuilt. Denial's root is in keeping one from having to face the pain of honest evaluation of one's self and behavior.

Having to admit that alcohol uses them instead of their using alcohol is most painful and humiliating. Often, the feeling of guilt and moral bankruptcy is at the root of all the alcohol-addicted person sees when looking in the mirror.

As is often the case, perspective is most important for the therapist who is irritated or angered by denial in an alcoholic's treatment. This therapist should give up, immediately, a lifetime habit. In giving up tobacco use, coffee and caffeine products, sweet products, fingernail biting, or whatever the substance may be, then the therapist learns two lessons. The first lesson is that the *addiction process is the same for all substances!* There is no difference in the addiction of the alcoholic and the addiction of the cigarette smoker. The second lesson is that no matter how much one may try, willpower is not enough and efforts will often fail at least once in the process. None of us are different in this process.

Thus, compassion and caring will be the approach to the alcoholic instead of anger and aggravation. Therapists' reluctance/refusal to diagnose alcohol abuse and alcohol addiction in others have roots in several important issues.

First, the clinician must examine and get in touch with personal attitudes toward any use of alcohol. A bottle of wine could be looked at by one and seen as a social companion and a substance that enhances special occasions; another may see the same bottle as wicked, sinful and harmful; another may see the bottle for use in religious ceremonies; still another may see the bottle as providing an acceptable escape from emotional pain. Each of these attitudes, and the incredible range between them, obviously color the willingness and ability of a therapist to deal with alcoholism.

Secondly, the therapist's own usage of alcohol-containing beverages is often significant. Alcoholism is not a respector of professional fields and therapists can slip into serious trouble with alcohol, which will limit any ability to deal with the question of alcohol usage in a client.

Thirdly is the unfinished business some therapists have because of alcohol abuse in their family, their friends or their coworkers. If, for example, the problems experienced by growing up in a home where one of the parents was an alcoholic are unresolved, the therapists will often be emotionally ill-equipped to deal with a family coming in for treatment.

Fourthly, the therapist is controlled by agency attitudes about diagnosing and treating alcoholism among the clientele. Some mental health agencies readily "program" their clinicians that alcohol use/abuse is a symptom of an underlying illness. Therefore, diagnosis should always reveal schizophrenia, depression, neurosis and a host of other problems, but never the alcohol use/abuse that brought the client into the center in the first place. Other clinics employ "specialists" to deal with alcohol clients, and none of the remaining staff pay much attention to this clientele. Often the remaining staff do not deal with these at all. Still other clinics provide workshop and in-services to equip the staff in diagnosing and treating the alcoholic and their significant others.

What all medical and psychological fields must understand is this: Minimally, one out of every nine persons in the continental United States who even takes one drink will become alcohol addicted at some point in their lives. Also, this problem of alcoholism diagnosis and treatment is the personal responsibility of every helping professional in the helping professions. The practice of licensed professionals, doctors, attorneys, psychiatrists, psychologists, counselors, social workers, nurses, educators, and those who comprise the clergy must include the ability to diagnose the alcohol addicted and their families. If for any of the reasons discussed above the diagnostician is unable to treat the affected persons, knowing who to refer them to is obligatory. Many professionals have closed their eyes to the pain and suffering of the alcoholic family system for much too long.

Therapists must be challenged to evaluate their knowledge and attitude towards clients who are suffering the devastation of alcoholism. If ten clients are evaluated and diagnosed and one of those is not suffering the effects of alcohol at some level, the clinician probably missed the diagnosis. Alcohol usage must be evaluated in every client. Between the one in ten who is addicted to alcohol, and the four of ten who are affected adversely by alcoholism in the family, this means five of every ten clients are probably in need of some form of alcoholism treatment and evaluation.

The problem is not going away because clinicians ignore the problem! In times of economic stress and hard times, divorce increases and alcoholism rates do also. Our capability to deal with these clients in an effective and humane way must also increase.

Sharon Wegscheider has identified keys to therapist effectiveness in her book, *Another Chance, Hope and Health for the Alcoholic Family*. These areas are vital to consider for all helping professionals.

The Whole Person Inventory*
(For Professionals)

This is not a standardized test, but a checklist of self-evaluation. The answers are not intended to yield a numerical score but rather a personal insight. There are no formal norms; the inventory reflects instead my observations of effectiveness, ineffectiveness, and burnout in a wide range of helping professionals throughout the country, who have attended my training workshops or work in the industrial or treatment programs for which I am a consultant.

S.W.

Physical Potential

Personal Life

— Take good care of my general health, including exercise, diet and rest.
— Enjoy using my body in sports, exercise, or dancing.
— Welcome sexuality as part of an an intimate relationship.
— Manage my time and energy to meet my own rather than someone else's priorities.
— Consider money primarily a resource for achieving my personal priorities.
— Consider my living and work environments as resources for enhancing my satisfaction in living.

Professional Life

— Provide a nurturing environment for treatment
— Maintain a balanced work load within the limitations of my work setting.
— Am alert for non-verbal communication in clients (facial expressions, posture, movements, tone of voice, etc.)
— Take a straightforward attitude about providing a service for which people pay.

Signs of Trouble

— Am often tired and lacking energy.
— Am eating, drinking, or smoking more than I feel I should.
— Tend to put off visiting the dentist and having health checkups.
— Am too busy or too tired to exercise regularly.
— Am often too busy to get away for a vacation.
— Use many of my vacations to attend professional workshops.

Emotional Potential

Personal Life

— Am in touch with my feelings

Professional Life

— Respect my client's feelings even

---

*From Sharon Wegscheider, *Another Chance,* 1981. Reprinted by permission of the author and publisher (Science & Behavior Books, Inc., Palo Alto, California 94306).

most of the time and respect them.
- Pay attention to my feelings as a necessary part of intuition.
- Give my feelings due weight in making decisions.
- Feel free and able to express my feelings in appropriate ways.
- Respect the feelings of others and their right to express them in appropriate ways.

though they differ from mine.
- Give clients permission to express their feelings in a safe atmosphere.
- Value my own feelings for what they can tell me about my client, our relationship, and the process.
- Respond to the client's deeper needs (as I see them) rather than reacting to his wishes or demands.
- Feel free to express my personal feelings to clients when doing so will not interfere with treatment goals.

Signs of Trouble

- Find that most of my clients have to work through similar feelings — often the same ones that I have to work through myself.
- Believe that a client's avowed feelings, when they do not fit my professional picture of his situation, are probably defensive.
- Expect clients to be able to get in touch with feelings promptly as they arise.
- Believe that showing concern for the client openly undermines the professional relationship.

Social Potential

Personal Life

- Am able to build and maintain satisfying relationships.
- Am open and honest with others, without fearing the consequences.
- Reveal my opinions and feelings without seeking others' approval.
- Am willing to be vulnerable in sharing information about myself.
- Am direct and honest in expressing my needs and wants.
- Am in control of how much or how little of myself I reveal and do so prudently.
- Am willing to do my part in maintaining relationships.

Professional Life

- Have a clear understanding of my relationship to my clients.
- Am honest with clients and with myself about what I can and cannot do.
- Make no promises about the outcome of treatment.
- Give the client my total attention while we are together.
- Can confront the behavior of a client while still supporting him as a person.
- Have a clear perception of my own life and history and of the part they play in the context of treatment.

Signs of Trouble

- Find making and maintaining eye contact uncomfortable.
- Find the demands of my work leaves little time for my family.

— Find the demands of my work leave little time for social activities.
— Spend most of my leisure time by myself.
— Spend most of my leisure time with others from my professional field or work setting.
— Tend to avoid discussing unpleasant topics with a client.
— Sometimes find myself making promises that I may not be able to keep.
— Discover sometimes that clients are embarrassed at the personal information about my life that I share with them.
— Sometimes find myself playing surrogate family member, friend, or lover to a client.

Mental Potential

Personal Life

— Am knowledgeable about many subjects.
— Enjoy learning new things and developing new skills.
— Can remember and acknowledge most events of my childhood including painful ones
— Am open and receptive to new ideas.
— Am imaginative in envisioning new alternatives.
— Know my limitations and do not hesitate to ask for information, suggestions, and help.

Professional Life

— Plan my work in an organized way.
— Am able to communicate clearly.
— Can remember previous sessions and recognize patterns.
— Can accept supervision and criticism.
— Make an active effort to keep informed about new developments in my field.
— Know my limitations and do not hesitate to refer a client to another professional.

Signs of Trouble

— Have little time to pursue hobbies or non-professional activities.
— Read mostly professional books and journals.
— Ten to use the same style of treatment with all clients.
— Try to fit clients into my theoretical model.
— Am cooly objective, feeling that it is more professional to see clients as cases rather than individual persons.
— Find I understand my clients so well that I often finish their sentences for them.
— Spend considerable time explaining my theoretical approach to my clients during treatment sessions.

Spiritual Potential

Personal Life

— Am convinced that life has meaning and direction.
— Am aware of some Power greater than myself.

Professional Life

— Feel a spirit of hope most of the time and communicate it to clients.
— Try to help each client see his

— Have a sense of my own relationship to the larger world, other people, and the Power greater than myself.
— Usually feel firmly balanced and grounded.
— Am aware that the roles I play in life are merely expressions of my true self.
— Feel accepting and accepted most of the time.

present pain in a wider context that also allows realistic hope.
— Help the client learn that he can feel responsible for his actions and yet acknowledge a reality greater than himself.
— Guide the client in his search for the true self beneath his roles.
— Can accept a client's choices for himself even when they differ from what I would choose for him.

Signs of Trouble

— Find the world a basically hostile place.
— Often feel that life is absurd and meaningless.
— Believe that I am totally responsible for whatever occurs in my life and that my client is responsible for his.
— Believe that outside forces control whatever occurs in my life and my clients, so we are in no way responsible.
— Consider "counselor" ("physician"), etc., as my basic identity.
— Find I am often critical of my friend's and client's values.
— Am convinced that my religion or spiritual path is the one true way and would convince my clients of this if I could.

Volitional Potential

Personal Life

— Am usually decisive even though I realize that I sometimes make mistakes.
— Am willing to take risks.
— Usually follow through on decisions with wholehearted action.
— Am disciplined and steady in whatever I undertake.
— Am persistent in the face of difficulty or discouragement.
— Can accept patiently such unavoidable frustrations as weather, physical limitations, and the idiosyncracies of people and institutions.

Professional Life

— Live up to the treatment contract I have made with the client.
— Expect the client to live up to the contract, too, doing his/her part according to his/her capabilities.
— Am willing to confront the client if he/she is not fulfilling the contract.
— Am willing to be directive when I feel the circumstances call for it.
— Am straightforward about my own needs and wants in the treatment relationship.
— Am responsible in routine matters such as punctuality, note-taking, and following institutional procedures.

Signs of Trouble

— Feel constantly overwhelmed with things that I cannot find time to do.
— Am habitually late for personal and professional appointments.

— Conform to schedules and rules rather than making my own choices.
— Find it very hard to say no.
— Find it hard to change my position once I have taken a stand.
— Believe a responsible counselor should be available to his/her clients whenever they wish to see him/her, without concern for his/her personal convenience.
— Believe that a counselor should not be expected to see clients outside regular appointments, regardless of the circumstances.
— Rarely offer my opinion and suggestions to friends or clients.
— Feel uncomfortable in setting and enforcing reasonable limits for my children, subordinates, or clients.
— Am strongly directive with clients and feel that failure to follow my directions should be seen as an unhealthy defense.

Chapter 3

DISEASE CONCEPT

Presentation of Concept

THE American Medical Association gave formal recognition to the disease concept of alcoholism in 1956. Since that time, numerous other treatment facilities have adopted this concept in treating the alcoholic. To classify a condition as a disease, it must be describable, predictable, progressive, of primary origin, permanent and potentially fatal.

Many programs teach the disease concept of alcoholism as the only valid method of alcoholism therapy. As with any approach, problems and flaws exist with this approach. However, the disease concept has enabled more people to be treated and to live sober, useful lives than any other approach to alcoholism treatment throughout history.

Old misconceptions and myths will always remain, but these are combatted quite effectively through education and through the recovery of persons who can go out and educate the public. Another problem with alcoholism as a disease is the number of people who are treated for alcoholism and don't experience sobriety as a result of that treatment. Rather than placing the responsibility on the drinker, the problem is often generalized in the approach used to treat the individual. Another problem in this process is that the chemically dependent person refuses to accept the disease concept, the spouses and families refuse to accept the disease concept and thus do not seek the treatment of hospital-based programs as early in the process as they could. Another dilemma in this process is that medical doctors, clergymen, psychiatrists, attorneys and other members of the professional community often refuse to diagnose alcoholism as an illness. Thus, if one of these individuals is consulted or becomes aware of the problem, they often become another enabler in the process of alcoholic addiction. The concept of an enabler is a person who, through ignorance, misconception, or their own struggle with alcoholism or alcoholism in a family member, is unable to deal with the disease as it presents itself and take therapeutic and helpful action for the individual. Thus, they enable the person to stay drunk.

Under AMA criteria, an illness can be described. Alcoholism can be described in terms of symptoms, in terms of diagnosis and in terms of behavior that goes with the process of becoming ill with this disease. The symptoms that can also be described in behavioral terms of this disease include a compulsion to drink. This means that despite every intention of having one drink and quitting, once a drink is taken the person can no longer control their destiny or what happens to them. Alcohol tolerance increases. Tolerance is defined as the increasing rate of metabolism of the alcohol, coupled with the decreasing impairment, despite a blood alcohol level that normally would indicate considerable intoxication. An example of this would be an individual with a blood alcohol level well above 0.20 who does not seem drunk, does not slur words, and can walk a reasonably straight line. This individual has increased tolerance to alcohol and is, at this point, addicted. How tolerance increases is not known; however, it is the nervous system's ability to adapt and function normally, despite the presence of alcohol in the bloodstream. Once tolerance increases, a person is guaranteed to go into withdrawal with a cessation of drinking; that is another key indication of the illness of alcohol.

Secondly, the course of the illness is predictable and progressive. Simply stated, this means that if treatment is not rendered for this disease, the person will get worse. As with many other diseases, a plateau in the process can occur. However, a plateau rarely lasts longer than a few months. The deterioration of this progressive illness acts on the physical, mental, and spiritual realm of the individual's life.

As the disease progresses, the person depends on alcohol more and more to do for them what they are unable to do for themselves. They become angry, hostile, and experience resentments they cannot even explain towards other persons. Often, the person refuses to discuss anything connected with their drinking or any of the obvious anxieties experienced as a result of drinking. The individual in the progression will lose interest in their family, their friends, their job (if they still have one) and any interests and hobbies that have been part of their lives for many years. The person may experience tremors and require an early morning drink. As the disease progresses, the periods of intoxication increase and the periods of sobriety decrease. The person will sincerely promise at different points to quit drinking, will be fully sincere in their efforts, and will fail repeatedly, causing further exhaustion of their excuses and further death of their self-respect. Near the final part of the drinking process, if treatment is not rendered, the person begins to deteriorate morally, in that they will commit acts they never even dreamed of committing. They neglect their food and nutritional requirements and subject their body organs to the repeated stress of alcohol intoxication, which results in physical deterioration. Sometimes, the physical deterioration also includes brain damage.

Further, if teatment is not rendered, death will result. Certainly the progressive nature of this disease and the predictability with which untreated alcoholics die should trigger more effort to get these people into treatment and to treat every aspect of this disease.

Third, the disease is primary. Most professionals for many years started from the premise that alcoholism was the symptom of whatever field it was that they represented. If the professional was a doctor, then alcoholism was treated as a disease that had a physical origin, and if this physical origin could be uncovered, the disease would disappear. Psychologists treated alcoholism as a symptom of an underlying anxiety, conflict, childhood difficulty, or characterological defect that once uncovered would arrest the alcoholism. Sociologists have come at it from an environmental approach. If the environment can be manipulated, then the individual no longer desires a drink. Repeatedly, the alcoholic was told "alcohol is not what's wrong with you, but we'll find out what it is and as soon as we find out what it is, we'll treat you and you will be alright." What this has produced for most alcoholics is considerable anxiety about what is wrong with them and emphasis on treating something that cannot even be defined, while the alcoholism that is killing them goes untreated. Alcoholism is a primary disease in and of itself — it's predictable, progressive and kills people. Because this is a primary disease, the disease causes (it's not the result of, but causes) mental, emotional and physical problems. For example, liver cirrhosis is a very serious illness, but liver cirrhosis cannot be treated unless the person becomes sober and stays sober. Depression, inability to cope, aging-related stresses, loss of income, and widowhood are serious mental problems in the elderly. They cannot be treated if the person comes to treatment sessions intoxicated.

Guilt, fear, grief, and loneliness are tremendous emotional problems of the elderly. These diffculties cannot be treated until the elderly alcoholic is sober. Alcoholism must be treated first if any of the other problems that plague this person are ever to be treated.

Fourth, the disease of alcoholism is permanent. Once a person is an alcoholic, they are always an alcoholic. They will always have an alcoholic response to drinking. The solution to alcoholism is abstinence, which means then the body, spirit, and mind can recover.

Alcoholics have to learn that they can never again return to a social drinking environment and maintain control of that drinking. Some alcoholics have stories about having achieved sobriety for ten, fifteen, or twenty years and, having decided that a drink of wine would not hurt them, they took that drink and no gross thing happened to them. So, a relatively short time later, they had another drink, but within a month everyone who has ever returned to the bottle has ended up on a binge. The progression of this disease continues whether the alcoholic is drinking or not.

The story of Mr. Jay is a perfect example of this. The man was fifty-seven years old and had been sober for fifteen years. At his son's wedding he allowed himself to have a drink of the champagne with the wedding toast; despite the concern of his family nothing terrible seemed to have happened to him. He had a drink, put it down, and left it alone. Mr. Jay shared with the treatment group the incessant craving that one drink caused in him. Three days later, he had two drinks. Two days after that, he binged, a binge that lasted six weeks and brought him into the hospital-based program semicomatose.

Despite fifteen years of sobriety, this client was not able to return to where he once was with his drinking, but his drinking illness picked up where it left off fifteen years earlier. The reaction was severe and almost cost the client his life. All treatment programs could document similar cases to this, and they occur frequently. Alcoholism is a chronic, permanent disease. Despite research that came out several years ago stating that the alcoholic could return to social drinking in some cases, the clinical evidence has said that this is not so, and even now those reports are being contradicted by the people who issued them.

Fifth, this is a terminal disease. If alcoholism remains untreated, the alcoholic will die a minimum of fifteen years sooner than he otherwise would have died. Further, life span can be shortened even more if accidental death is alcohol related.

The terminal alcoholic also often kills (not knowingly but just as dead) innocent people that are involved in his path. This can be boating accidents, fires, and most often, auto accidents. Those who write death certificates use a lot of euphemism in alcoholism cases and would much rather write down that the person had a heart attack, died of high blood pressure, a liver disorder or some other cause, instead of writing that the person died of an alcohol related death.

This has made the urgency of the problem seem less real even to those providing alcohol treatment. This is a drug that precipitates slow, painful, and often isolated death, especially for the elderly alcoholic. These five components have resulted in the disease concept being taught virutally in a universal fashion now.

Pros

There have been several tremendous advantages to the disease concept.

Firstly, it has allowed persons to come into treatment and receive treatment with a third-party reimbursement. This has been especially important to someone on a limited income, such as an elderly individual.

Secondly, it has allowed hospital-based programs to get a footing and be available to a wider range of people than some of the more exclusive types of programs were.

Thirdly, the employed alcoholic can now use sick leave, can check into a hospital program and can receive medical, nutritional and alcohol treatment at the same time while not having to face the consequences of losing their job because of a non-medical absence.

Fourthly, the disease process has enabled families to begin receiving the treatment that they require, without the stigma of the moral weakness argument that was so often applied to the family. Certainly, no one will take it upon themselves to condem the wife of a diabetic who went to the hospital to participate in learning how to administer and understand the insulin her husband takes or to understand the diet that was required and how to adapt foods to the new life-style.

Certainly, alcoholism programs have enjoyed tremendous success in treating families of the alcoholic with a similar approach. The family members are told, "This disease has affected you, it has affected your family, and here's what we can do to help you, as a family, recover." The exciting thing about this process is that it has enabled families to recover, even when the alcoholic did not.

Cons

For all the good the disease concept has done in the field and in getting these persons into treatment and keeping them there, the disease concept itself has some serious drawbacks. Unfortunately, one of these has been that alcoholism has been a word that has not been completely understood in all its entirety. That alcoholism is killing people is something that is not talked about with the conviction that needs to be there. Alcoholism does not carry the emotional impact of the words *alcohol addiction*. As the Do It Now Foundation points out, "alcohol addiction was much too harsh and linked too much reality to the alcoholic's true situation.

It is about time that we started greater public awareness about alcoholism as a harmful chemical, not simply a popular mystique as it seems to have become in many circles" (Pawlak, Frazier, and Gray, 1975).

While the disease concept has enabled significant numbers of persons to recover from alcoholism, this concept has produced a misunderstanding of the relationship of alcohol addiction to other addictions. This has been especially harmful in the treatment of cross-addicted poly drug users.

A heroin addict who battles through this addiction and then becomes addicted to alcohol is taught contradictory information. The person as a heroin addict is told the problem is primarily a physiological addiction with resulting emotional and social consequences. Then, when entering an alcoholism treatment program, they are taught the problem is a special disease that has special components.

The fact is that the addiction process is the same regardless of what substance a person is addicted to. The process theory of addiction helps poly drug users to solve the *how* of the addiction. Addiction theory also resolves many of the issues over which professionals argue. No addict dares to return to the substance usage unless desiring readdiction. This is true of opiates, tobacco, alcohol, caffeine and similar substances. The mystery is solved immediately as to cause.

Heavy usage of any drug or substance, over a long enough period of time, results in dependence and withdrawal symptoms when withdrawn. Alcoholism and heavy social drinking are not different in the economic, social and familial difficulties encountered. Many heavy social drinkers die the same types of death as the alcoholic. Some have pointed to those individuals who drink one time and have adverse reaction. This issue is one of an allergic reaction to a drug, not instant alcoholism. An allergic reaction to a substance occurs in every pharmaceutical class.

The process theory also solves the issue of when a heavy drinker becomes an alcoholic. If a heavy drinker incurs the consequences and stops or cuts back on drinking, then alcoholism is stopped. This phenomenon has caused some of the literature to discuss alcohol abuse in terms of problem drinkers rather than alcoholic.

The process theory solves the issue of "why me." The answer is that the person drank enough to become addicted. Once addicted, all the implications discussed under the disease concept are applicable. An individual cannot become an alcoholic unless the person drinks enough ethanol to become one. The alcoholic personality has never been successfully proven because many persons who don't drink act and think the same way. Conversely, many alcohol-addicted persons never manifest the so-called alcoholic personality.

To quote Pawlak, Frazier, and Gray:

> The disease concept in itself is now and probably always will be an extremely valid one. But it is only one good concept — the tip of the iceberg — among others which are needed today to develop a total viewpoint — especially concerning the area of education to the consequences of alcohol use on all social and personal levels. No longer can we afford to be so selective regarding whom we are trying to reach. No longer can we afford to ignore educating people on the simple facets of alcohol which can have so many ramifications regarding such things as pregnancy, accidental overdoses, from combinations with other common drugs, and vitamin deficiencies which lead to serious disease and other complications.

Regardless of what concept is used, certain indicators or symptoms signal the progression of an individual into increasingly serious difficulty. In Chapter 2, the full chart is presented with de-escalation into the process and re-escalation towards total recovery.

Chapter 4

ASSESSMENT OF ALCOHOLISM
IN THE GENERAL POPULATION

Background

ONE major reason for lack of assessment for alcoholism among institutionalized patients is helping professions failing to grasp the magnitude of the problem. When patients die in hospitals due to alcohol withdrawal, which is undiagnosed, the tragedy is compounded.

Mr. K was seventy-four years old when a wart on his foot began to change. His wife persuaded him to consult a doctor, who diagnosed a localized cancer that was to be removed by surgery. Upon hospital admission, he was asked by his nurse if he drank alcohol-containing beverages. "Oh, you know, one glass of wine with my spaghetti." Following the administering of the anesthetic, the patient went into complete arrest. He died without regaining consciousness.

Despite the onset of withdrawal symptoms (jitteryness, cold sweats, tremors), his alcoholism was not diagnosed. The symptoms of his withdrawal were attributed to pre-surgery anxiety. Once further depressing drugs were administered to this alcoholic male, the brain shut itself down and the person died.

If cases such as this were rare, one could look the other way. These cases are not isolated. Many patients die in hospitals each year in America because of lack of assessment.

One easy method of assessing these patients is to require a

blood alcohol level as part of every admission workup. Due to the denial and fear of most alcoholics, these individuals do not give accurate answers to questions on alcohol consumption. Remember, the higher the BAL without signs of intoxication, the higher the probability that the individual is an addicted drinker. This same kind of embarrassment has led most hospitals to do a VDRL blood test for venereal disease as a matter of routine. Thus, embarrassing questions regarding sexual activity are not asked, but any VD is diagnosed and can be treated.

Utilizing the blood alcohol level test in this manner will identify alcoholism in a cost-effective and non-offensive manner. Further, once identified, this test can be used to confront the patient as to use of alcohol and the treatment indicated.

Since many patients are admitted with physiological conditions resulting from alcohol abuse, assessment must be completed or the physician becomes an enabler.

Statistically, the prevalence of alcoholism in male patients in general hospitals ranges from 25 percent to 30 percent (Reading, 1974). The incidence in Veterans Administration hospital studies has found this percentage as high as 55.3 percent (Funkhouser, 1978).

In psychiatric wards, the percentages are equally distressing. Simon (1968) evaluated 534 admissions to the San Francisco General Hospital. Of these admissions, 23 percent were alcoholic.

McCuster, Cherubin and Zimberg (1971) conducted a survey in Harlem of adults age 50 to 69. They discovered 63 percent of the males and 34 percent of the females were alcoholic.

Routine laboratory assessment can also indicate a probability of alcohol abuse. A report by Funkhouser (1978) showed the following systemic studies of alcoholics:

Test	Level	Percentage of Cases
WBC	High	69
HCT	Low	85
Uric Acid	High	89
Total Protein	Low	42

Further, the alcoholic will test low for potassium and magnesium, which will produce cardiac difficulties. Dietary distress is also evident in alcoholics, some who cannot tolerate food due to periods of prolonged drinking.

Self-Report Questionnaire

Other assessment tools are available to facilitate diagnosis of the disease. In 1977, the state of Florida published the following assessment tool.

1. You can only become an alcoholic by drinking (a) hard liquor (b) wine (c) beer (d) any alcoholic beverage.
2. Alcohol is the most widely used drug in America. True or False?
3. Most people who become alcoholics (a) drink alcoholic beverages (b) have personality disorders (c) deny their illness (d) use alcohol as an escape (e) all are correct.
4. Anyone who must drink in order to function or to "cope" with life has a severe drinking problem. True or False?
5. Alcohol is a stimulant. True or False?
6. Most alcoholics are on skid row. True or False?
7. There are certain symptoms to warn people that their drinking may be leading to alcoholism. True or false?
8. Anyone who by his own personal definition, or that of his family and friends, frequently drinks to a state of intoxication has a drinking problem. True or False?
9. Alcoholism is treatable. True or False?
10. Heavy drinking and drunkenness are the same as alcoholism. True or False?
11. Occasional social drinking is not apt to damage the tissues or heart, kidneys, or brain. True or False?
12. Anyone who goes to work intoxicated has a drinking problem. True or False?
13. Absenteeism may be a clue to an alcoholic employee in industry. True or False?
14. The suicidal rate amongst alcoholics is very high. True or False?

15. Alcohol-related offenses account for this percentage of all U.S. arrests reported annually. (a) 10% (b) 25% (c) 50% (d) 80%
16. Anyone who is intoxicated while driving a car has a drinking problem. True or False?
17. You can have an alcoholic around you and not be aware of it. True or False?
18. Anyone who sustains a bodily injury which requires medical attention as a consequence of an intoxicated state has a drinking problem. True or False?
19. A person has to consume alcoholic beverages daily to be classified as an alcoholic. True of False?
20. Anyone who comes into conflict with the law as a consequence of an intoxicated state has a drinking problem. True or False?
21. To sober up (a) drink black coffee (b) take a cold shower (c) jog (d) let time pass.
22. Loss of judgment and the ability for self-criticism occur before there are obvious symptoms of intoxication. True or False?
23. Alcohol is a member of the anesthetic series of drugs. True or False?
24. Anyone who, under the influence of alcohol, does something he vows he would never do without alcohol has a drinking problem. True or False?
25. Alcohol is a mood modifier. True or False?

Answers

1. d	7. T	13. T	19. F
2. T	8. T	14. T	20. T
3. e	9. T	15. c	21. d
4. T	10. F	16. T	22. T
5. F	11. T	17. T	23. T
6. F	12. T	18. T	24. T
			25. T

Assessment of Intoxication, Withdrawal, and Chronic Syndromes

Intoxication Syndromes

Simple Intoxication. Slurred speech, staggering gait, dilated pupils, and slow rate of pulse and respiration may be present. Feelings of guilt, depression, or hostility may be present. Some emotional liability may be present. Referral to detox is certainly appropriate if medical status permits.

Pathological Intoxication. The onset of this disorder is dramatic and sudden, typically after *minimal amounts* of alcohol intake (often as little as one or two drinks). The patient is confused, disoriented, and experiences illusions, delusions and visual hallucinations. The patient will be hyperactive and agitated, typically impulsive and aggressive. Rage, anxiety, and depression are typical emotional components. Hospitalization is indicated for maximal management of the patient.

Acute Intoxication. This is an acute brain syndrome of psychotic proportions that is brought on by alcohol intake in much *greater* quantities than the pathological intoxication type mentioned above. Also, rule out alcoholic hallucinosis and DT's. Hospitalization is indicated.

Alcoholic Paranoia. This is typically reported as a vague sense of discomfort, suspiciousness and mistrust of others. Often, these patients are aware that these sensations/beliefs are not real and can sometimes relate the onset of such ideas to a recent change in drinking pattern. Patients often report delusions of reference, associating overhead conversations or sounds to themselves. Such delusions are not commonly well formulated or well developed, but on occasion may be elaborate.

Withdrawal Syndromes

Mild Withdrawal. Mild withdrawal symptoms begin six to seven hours after the last drink or after a radical reduction in alcohol intake. Patient experiences tremulousness (the "shakes"), weakness, profuse perspiration and high anxiety level. Also, patients will complain of "shaking inside" when obvious motor disturbance may not be present. Headache, nausea, anorexia, and vomiting may be present. Patient may also be hyperreflexive and will startle easily.

Alcoholic Hallucinosis. The peak time for this to occur is twenty-four hours after last drink. Patient may report any and all types of hallucinations in varying combinations. Often the patient will experience such hallucinations in a vague, erratic manner. Common complaints are occasional musical sounds, tones, or noises, odd visceral sensations (i.e. crawling, itching, tingling), and visual patterns of vague light flashes and/or shapeless objects. Snakes, maggots, bugs and elephants are also common visual hallucinations. This may begin when patient's eyes are closed, but over time will continue when eyes are open. Alcoholic hallucinosis may precede the onset of DT's.

Delerium Tremens. This may occur from one to ten days after last drink. Usually onset is within forty-eight to seventy-two hours. Psychotic symptomatology (disorientation in any and all three spheres, hallucinations, delusions) as well as physical components are present. Patient will be quite agitated at times and quite restless. Erratic and/or rapid pulse rate as well as elevated blood pressure usually accompany this syndrome. Hospitalization is indicated with a diagnosis of DT's, impending DT's, or acute withdrawal syndrome.

Be aware that intoxication/withdrawal syndromes vary among individuals. Delerium tremens, hallucinosis, paranoia and seizures may *all* occur, may occur in any combination, or may not occur at all. Any identified seizure patient should be hospitalized immediately and medicated accordingly. Delerium tremens is a medical emergency.

Chronic Syndromes

Alcoholic Deterioration. This chronic brain syndrome presents a similar clinical picture to other forms of the organic brain syndrome (OBS). At first glance, the patient may appear reasonably intact. Patient will evidence subtle memory impairment, impaired judgment and some disorientation. Some confabulation may be present, but to moderate levels. *Concrete* thinking is very common.

Korsakoff's Syndrome. Amnesia, a high degree of confabulation and disorientation to time and place are present. Acute impairment of immediate memory is common. In addition, physiological conditions are present, especially peripheral neuropathy. Although this is often labeled OBS, the proper medical diagnosis should be made.

Wernicke's Syndrome. This condition is due to vitamin and other nutritional deficiencies commonly found as a result of chronic alcoholism. Beginning with delerium, it consists of paralysis of one or more of the optic motor nerves (ophthalmoplegia), memory loss, confabulation, apathy, ataxia, and at times coma. This condition is relatively rare and not to be confused with Korsakoff's.

Polyneuropathy. This neurological disorder is typically a result of vitamin and nutritional deficiencies, as well as electrolyte imbalance associated with chronic alcoholism. However, this condition may be present in addition to or in the absence of other disorders. It typically manifests itself in the lower extremities but may progress to the upper limbs. Diagnosis is difficult if head trauma, diabetes, or stroke are present.

Polyneuropathy is experienced by the patient as a sensation of tingling and weakness, as well as some loss of coordination and gross motor control in the calf and thigh muscles.

Other complications in diagnosing alcoholism revolve around the alcoholic who self-medicates serious psychiatric and physical disorders. While some physicians treat this as a form of denial, this is a valid cause of addiction.

Arthritis, back injury, pain from broken hips and other causes of acute pain are often medicated by alcohol consumption. After all, this "medication" is inexpensive and does not require a physician or pharmacist. Particularly at risk for this process are the poor elderly who cannot afford appropriate medical care.

When such an individual is seen in the emergency room, the physician often does only a cursory examination and then refers to detoxification and/or psychiatric personnel. Thus, appropriate care is not given.

Most alcoholism treatment staffs can cite cases where an alcoholic was dried out only to present severe psychiatric symptomatology. Since alcohol depresses anxiety and many forms of psychotic process, the patient begins to use alcohol to "feel better." Again, alcohol is inexpensive and does not require psychiatrists and mental health involvement.

Other mental health concerns that facilitate alcoholism are grief, depression, loneliness and boredom. The time has come to cease paying "lip service" to the treatment of alcoholism. The alcoholic requires the same urgent, courteous treatment given other serious illnesses.

Diagnostic Tips

1. Be direct and frank when discussing the patient's illness. The patient will notice uncertainty and be less likely to give a positive result.
2. Ask direct, open-ended questions. This makes evasive answers much more difficult to give.
3. Accept the patient as he/she is. Give the individual unconditional regard.
4. Help the patient understand that this illness occurs and to concentrate on getting well first. "Why" is the unanswerable question.
5. Realize that denial is part of the process of alcoholism; do not be angered by the patient's denial of alcoholism. When a physician diagnoses cancer, denial is often the response too.
6. Allow the patient to ventilate the emotions as they experience them. Even though the physician is also human, he/she cannot be therapeutic if caught up in the anger, pain and hostility that is expressed.
7. The stronger the denial that alcohol is a problem, the more the probability the person is in serious difficulty with drinking.
8. Be familiar with community resources for the treatment of alcoholism. Make referral as appropriate.
9. Do not give any prescription for tranquilizers, sedative hypnotics, or other drugs. The person must learn to deal with life without chemical assistance.

Chapter 5

MEDICAL AND PHYSICIAN'S ISSUES

Systems Review

ONCE a physician has admitted a patient verified to have alcoholism, certain exams become vitally important. In this chapter, some of those systems and possible effects and observations that the physician can make will be outlined.

While not all alcoholics will be affected in every system by their disease, it is nonetheless important that the doctor examine the patients from head to toe and determine what effects the person has undergone and what remedial treatment is required. While psychotherapy alcoholism inpatient treatment and a variety of other approaches might be desirable and recommended, statistics indicate that it is vitally important that the alcoholic be medically treated. The treatment should include all that is wrong with him. Once the treatment is complete, any other psychotherapy or alcoholism therapy that is undertaken will be more meaningful.

Logically, the more one feels good, the more one will benefit from such strategies. Thus, the systems review is vitally important. Initially, the skin should be examined. Five percent of all alcohol that enters the body goes through the skin. As a drying agent, the water is pulled out of the cells and causes dehydration. Dehydration for an elderly alcoholic can be a life-threatening situation. Other skin observations that may be noticed are bruises, which may indicate falls, cigarette burns from not being able to carefully put out a cigarette once it is lit, and contusions which may or may not be realized by the patient initially. Another skin observation that can be vitally important is that of vascular spidal anguma. This unusual pigmentation is caused by vitamin B deficiency, which indicates liver disease. Should this be present, again, remedial efforts are vitally important.

The next area for evaluation should be the cranial area. It is a well-known fact that many alcoholics, when intoxicated, fall but do not remember that they have fallen and thus can have serious head injuries that may not be diagnosed or treated. Additionally, because of the offense of the intoxication, many alcoholics who have serious head injuries are not evaluated properly because the dizziness, disorientation, dilation of the pupils and other indications of head injury are attributed to the intoxicated state. Many alcoholics die in this country every year following emergency room treatment because such injuries are not diagnosed or evaluated. Some of the cranial observations that might be noted are large bumps on the head. In an elderly person, all of these become vitally important, particularly any indication of bleeding. Since the elderly at large are more at risk for stroke to begin with, any kind of cranial swelling, discoloring, or other observable symptoms needs to be carefully evaluated. Another observation that can be made concerning the cranial area is whether or not the client complains of pain as the alcohol wears off. Again, it may be several days into the detoxification process before this criteria is really helpful being that withdrawal can cause a headache. Another cranial observation is whether there is puffiness and deep lines around the eyes; whether there is vascular or pallor engorgement. Such an observation can indicate other system dysfunction as well as dysfunction in the cranial area.

One of the best indicators of complications regarding alcoholism shows up through eye exams. Again, this is logical considering the amount of vitamin A that alcohol depletes in the system of any alcoholic, particularly that of an elderly alcoholic. The physician should be very aware that a lack of vitamin A causes night blindness and not be trapped into believing that the night blindness is a result of old age rather than alcohol intake and abuse. Several observations concerning the eyes can be immediately helpful in the diagnosis and treatment of alcoholism. For example, the pupil size and reaction is a good indicator of whether drugs are being used, particularly alcohol. Either pinpoint or wide pupil size and reaction is indicative of drug use. If the pupils are either but different in size from each other, it indicates a neurological problem and the cranial area should be examined more carefully. Pale conjunctiva indicates anemia. This is present in approximately 95 percent of all elderly alcoholics due to the vitamin deficiency and the inability to keep their food down as the alcoholism progresses. This must be immediately treated if health is to be restored. The internal visual exam can indicate high blood pressure and/or diabetes, both of which are vital in dealing with the general health and well-being of the elderly alcoholic. This is particularly important in the black elderly: the yellow sclera indicates hepatitis and/or sclerosis. This exam must be conducted without artificial light, as artificial light can hide the yellow tint of the eye and cause the clinician who checks for this to miss it. Also, if a sustained nystagmus is present in the eyes (rhythmic oscillations), it indicates a neurological problem, and a neurological workup should be completed immediately.

The neurological system cannot be adequately examined under the offense of alcohol. The clinician would do well to remember that alcohol both sedates and irritates all of the neurological system, particularly the central nervous system. Neurological problems may even occur before alcoholism is suspected, because alcoholics frequently have a decreased food intake and an increased liver disease. The decreased food intake is particularly evident in elderly alcoholics upon initial examination. Thus, a treatment program becomes doubly important not only for the treatment of the alcoholism itself but as a way of detaining and treating the anemia, dehydration and vitamin deficiencies that the elderly alcoholic has. If it is an economically deprived elderly individual, this is also doubly important since they usually cannot afford all that is necessary to restore good physical health. Also, the problem of the neurological system exam taken of the individual while under intoxication is that it is difficult to be sure what disease or condition is responsible for each of the symptoms noted. Thus, rarely can an accurate neurological exam be completed until after the person is detoxified for at least three or four days.

Some observations on the initial neurological exam, particularly if done in the emergency room, might be helpful for the doctor. First of all, what is his general status? If the person is intoxicated but alert, a mental status exam is appropriate. The mood, the affect and whether or not the person is hallucinating are vital in this category. Thirdly, what is the motor status of the individual? Is there ataxia present? Is the person slow, shuffling, short stepped, standing with a wide base stance? Are there tremors or paralysis present? Again, this is a very difficult exam to conduct in the elderly because very likely there's slowness of gait anyway due to age. This exam is best done if there is a member of the family or friend present who knows the person and can tell the clinician whether the motor status exam is due to the alcohol intake at present or whether the person is like this when they are sober. If memory can be tested (and this depends on the degree of intoxication), confabulation is an important component of this exam. Also, under the neurological system it is very important to find out if the person has ever had an epileptic seizure or been diagnosed an epileptic. Also important to determine is whether the seizures take place when intoxicated or when withdrawing from alcohol, because seizures are going to occur the first twelve to forty-eight hours in the elderly, usually as the brain detoxifies from the alcohol. Also important under the neurological exam is whether blackouts have occurred. Remember to explain to the family that a blackout is that the person has walked, talked and acted, then several hours later is unable to remember the incidents being described for them. Perhaps a case history here would be helpful.

Mr. D was a seventy-two year-old alcoholic who had been sober for some ten years but due to some situational stress returned to drinking. After the third night of drinking, he came home and proceeded to pick a fight with his wife and then struck his wife several times on the face, resulting in a black eye and a bruised cheekbone for his wife. She called the police, who brought him to the emergency room for evaluation. After three days of hospitalization, the staff and the wife confronted this alcoholic on his injury to his wife. He was astonished and could not understand that he had done this and could not believe he was responsible. She immediately accused him of always being like this when he was drinking and then denying that he had hurt her.

History showed that the man was, in fact, acting in a blackout and did not have any knowledge of his actions, what he did, or where he had been even though several people were able to describe his behavior during this time. Another important point under the neurological exam is that if the person is prone to have seizures during the withdrawal, some combination of Dilantin®, a sedative, may be appropriate during the withdrawal phase, so that the client does not go into seizures and possibly die during this time.

The next major system requiring a careful evaluation is that of the cardiovascular system. Alcohol inflames the heart when taken in large quantities. This inflammation will show up on an EKG as well as a chest x-ray. The percentage of coronary heart disease increases with alcohol intake about 2.5 ounces and decreases below 2.5 ounces consumed per day. In an elderly alcoholic, this again becomes a primary concern due to age-related changes in the heart, particularly if diabetes, arteriosclerosis or heart disease has been confirmed either in the patient or the patient's family history. There are several observable heart conditions that can suggest in reverse that the patient may in fact be in some trouble with alcohol. Any EKG change in the T wave of the EKG suggests heart difficulty that may be, in fact, alcohol related.

Also, there is a so-called "holiday heart" syndrome, which are those that show up in emergency rooms between Sunday and Tuesday after a weekend of drinking with fibrillations in their EKG patterns. These normally change after some period of detoxification has elapsed. The ones that do not change after detox are those with alcoholic cardiomyopathy. This is the inflammation of the heart due to fatty tissue forming because of the alcohol which does not return back to normal after abstinence of some period of time. These persons must, especially in the elderly category, be warned that if they drink again, they will, in fact, have a fatal heart attack. Again, the heart is one of the major organs that is stressed in any period of detoxification. If any history of heart difficulties shows up either in the patient's family or in the patient himself careful monitoring during any detoxification regimen that is undertaken, whether in a detox unit or in a general hospital ward, is suggested.

Moving from the cardiovascular system into the respiratory system again shows that the lungs are affected very obviously by prolonged alcohol abuse. This is, again, particularly true for the elderly alcoholic whether the person has just become an alcoholic or whether the person has been an alcoholic for a number of years. At least 10 percent of what is consumed is expelled through the lungs. Some current research suggest that some of the lung cancers associated with smoking may, in fact, be carcinoma caused by prolonged alcohol abuse. One confirmed effect of alcohol on the lungs is that of impairing the protective mechanism in the airways of the bronchia and the ventillatory function of the lungs themselves. During post-intoxication treatment, it is important to monitor the general breathing pattern to determine whether or not this is impaired. The sedative effect of alcohol on the respiratory system, particularly in the general alcohol population after 200 over 100 milliliters or in the elderly as low as 150 over 100 milliliters blood alcohol concentration, suggests that it can shut down due to the sedation of the brain and the lungs. So, the key is the higher the blood alcohol concentration in the core of the person's general health, the more closely the respiratory system must be monitored during post-drinking treatment.

The next area of great impairment for the alcoholic is that of the gastrointestinal system. The reason for this is that alcohol irritates the stomach and duodenal area of the colon. Ninety-five percent of the alcohol consumed by any individual is absorbed through these membranes. The liver is a primary site for detoxification, and the irritation leads to eventual blockage and accumulation of dead cells in the liver as it becomes fatty, inflamed and scarred (sclerosis). The pancreas also becomes irritated, and the passage of digestive chemicals can also become blocked here. As the enzymes start to accumulate, the pancreas begins to digest itself causing the lining to break down. This is called hemorrhagic pancreatitis. Once this has occurred, the alcoholic who drinks again will have another attack, guaranteed. This is one of the most painful of all infirmities that the alcoholic bears. Added to the pancreatitis is the misfunction of the insulin-producing regulator in the pancreas, which can shoot an alcoholic into a diabetic coma very, very quickly. Both the central organs of the body as well as the blood sugar level have to be monitored if the person has a pancreatitis attack. Unfortunately, this is the most difficult of all the exams that the doctor has to perform because of the overlap of the organs and the organs being enclosed in the abdominal cavity (see Fig. 5-1). Some general guidelines for the doctors might be in order.

SYSTEMS REVIEW AND LOCATION

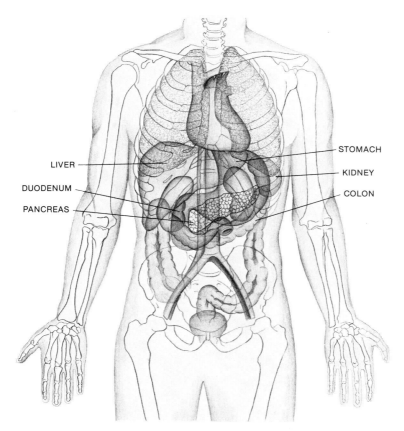

Figure 5-1. A quick review of the location and relation of the organs most damaged by alcohol abuse can be seen.

PATHOLOGY OF STOMACH

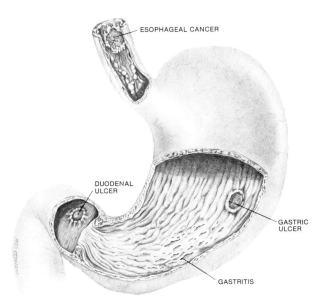

Figure 5-2. This composite of stomach pathologies demonstrates the tissue damage inflicted on this organ by repeated drinking episodes.

PATHOLOGY OF LIVER

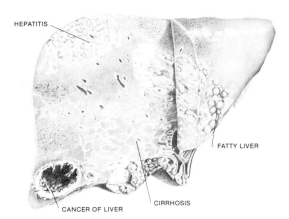

Figure 5-3. This composite demonstrates the major pathologies of the liver. While some of these can occur apart from alcoholism, alcohol abuse must be evaluated carefully when any of these conditions are present.

First, if the associated conditions are in the stomach and the intestines alone as shown in Figure 5-2, a heartburn-type syndrome is usually seen after a booze binge and the person will be regurgitating hydrochloric acid from the stomach. Likewise, there is blood in the stool during this period also. This person is also very likely to complain frequently of pain regardless of what is eaten during the first days of reintroducing food into this person's life-style. If the problem is in the liver, then the abdominal area will be enlarged with no tenderness indicating a fatty liver (see Fig. 5-3). If the abdominal area is enlarged with a smooth tender edge, then this indicates hepatitis, which can be deadly in a very short period of time for an elderly person. This person should be treated as a major medical emergency and given appropriate priority. An enlarged abdomen with a large, smooth, nontender edge indicates cirrhosis. To verify cirrhosis, the doctor should listen with his stethoscope for a venus hum indicative of an increase in collateral circulation. Also, ascites can be observed by the contour of the abdomen. Fluid goes to the lowest point and produces bulging plains, and if the patient is turned on his side, the fluid shifts accordingly. Cirrhosis is also a condition that does not improve but will stabilize and remain stable if the person abstains from alcohol over a long period of time. To diagnose pancreas problems, the symptomatology includes nausea and vomiting and is accompanied by epigastric tenderness. This epigastric pain may be severe enough for the patient to collapse as it radiates to the lumbar region and up into the left shoulder. To differentiate from heart attack and pancreas involvement requires an EKG and a careful examination. Also, the pancreas area can be palpitated and epigastric tenderness noted. Any rebounding of the abdominal wall i.e. (Is it soft with no muscle rigidity?) will verify the diagnosis of pancreatitis (see Fig. 5-4).

The next organ system that must be carefully evaluated is that of the kidney and bladder, or the urinary tract system. This is due in part to the fact that a great deal of all alcohol that is consumed is expelled through the kidneys and bladder. Prolonged abuse of alcohol will cause the kidneys to dump albumin until the anti-diuretic hormone of the brain takes over, causing fluid accumulation and a swelling of the kidney area. This is an extremely

PATHOLOGY OF PANCREAS

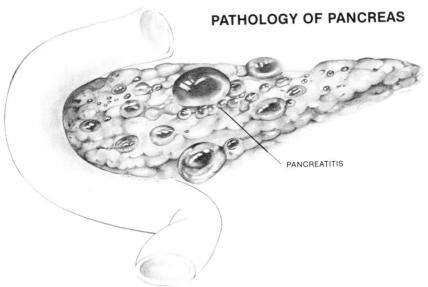

PANCREATITIS

Figure 5-4. Pancreatitis is the most painful of conditions and will often re-occur with each drinking episode following onset.

painful condition, and a diuretic pill that is given for this will only add to the problem. This patient requires hospitalization and natural diuretics such as herbs to deal with the problem. The bladder can also stretch, causing frequency of urination and a constant feeling of the person needing to urinate whether they do or not. If the urethra is also involved, it can cause a backup of the urine into the urinary tract, causing a serious and life-threatening infection.

There are two simple diagnostic tests that can be done with the urine, however, that can indicate the possibility of alcohol-related disease in the liver. First, the color of the urine is important. If urine is shaken in a test tube and it foams yellow then this indicates that liver disease is present. The second test is one to see if bile is present. Also, if the urine is dark colored, dehydration is present. This may also indicate a serious infection in the urinary tract and should be carefully investigated with the appropriate tests. Any problems in the urinary tract can likewise cause problems in the genital area of either the man or woman alcoholic.

For the female, vaginal lubrication decreases, causing painful and damaging intercourse with a man, if attempted at all. For the man, the testosterone decrease causes the testicles to decrease to half size, scrotal edema, and an inability to obtain or keep an erection. If the prostate is also experiencing some swelling, this will cause considerable difficulty for a man in attempting to empty his bladder and maintain an erection The breast area of the female and male both changes with increasing liver dysfunction due to the hormal changes that occur. Males will experience an increase in fatty breast tissue, often disproportionate to the rest of their body. Women will experience decrease in breast tissue, often also smaller than her body size would suggest.

The other system that will indicate important problems for the elderly is that of the hematopoietic system. The characteristics of these difficulties include clumps of red blood cells, which slows the circulation and decreases oxygen to the brain. Otherwise healthy people who experience strokes may be experiencing them due to this problem. It also slows the white blood cells' ability to engulf and destroy, thereby increasing their susceptibility to the common cold, viral infections and other bacterial infections. Either of the two blood counts that indicate this problem must become a differential diagnosis in determining if alcohol is causing this problem or if any of a number of other problems could also be indicated. Also, of major concern in elderly clients, particularly, is a destruction that alcohol causes to the platelets, which increases bleeding and bruising, coupled with a suppression of bone marrow, which, of course, is what produces blood. The outcome of these effects, of course, is that the alcoholic who falls or is otherwise cut will bleed easier and for a longer period of time. Thus, all of the interventions that are appropriate for those hemophiliac patients should also be employed at this point with the elderly alcoholic who is experiencing these changes.

Management of Withdrawal

Withdrawal from alcohol is a major medical crisis that requires medical care (see Fig. 5–1). If a detoxification unit is not available, then the person should be hospitalized in a medical ward for treatment.

Every detoxification unit has some form of standing orders that are administered automatically when a patient is admitted. In a community without deltox units, a given medical ward needs to be designated and standing orders must be initiated!

The physicians must decide their personal preferences for medications to combat each of the physical effects of withdrawal. Since psychiatric symptoms are also prevalent, each community must decide how to best meet the client's need.

But each emergency worker must know what the procedure is. At no time must these very ill people be bounced about without being admitted and treated.

Table 5-I

WITHDRAWAL STATES

	Mild	Moderate	Severe
Mental States:			
Thought content	Intact and fully oriented	Mild confusion — usually to date/time	Marked confusion and disorientation
Thought process	No hallucinations Able to converse	Often vague, illusions (at night) Mild visual and auditory hallucinations	Severe visual hallucinations; sense of danger related to hallucinations Suicide possible
Sleep	Restless sleep/mild insomnia	Marked insomnia some nightmares	Total insomnia
Appetite	Impaired/often eats only with medication	Marked impairment Generally drinks fluids only	Often rejects all food and fluids May require IV
Mood	Mildly depressed	Marked depression	Often depressed, paranoid and at times violent
Anxiety	Mild restlessness Some pacing	Marked restlessness; unable to sit or lie any period of time	Extreme restlessness and agitated
Psychomotor Activity	Inner shaking feelings with some hand tremors	Visible hand tremors and fine body shakes	Gross, uncontrolled body shaking

(*Table 5-1 continued*)

Physical States:

	Mild	Moderate	Severe
Blood pressure	Normal or slightly elevated systolic	Usually elevated systolic	Elevated systolic and diastolic
Pulse	Tachycardia	Pulse 100-120	Pulse 120-140
Nausea	Nauseous – able to drink fluids	Nausea and vomiting, not able to drink fluids without medication	Dry heaves and vomiting/rejects all fluids
Dehydration	Minimal or absent	Moderate	Severe
Muscular condition	Mild soreness	Soreness and cramps	Tenderness, cramps twitching
Sweating	Mostly during day	Some sweating both day and night	Severe loss of body fluids both day and night
Convulsion	Most infrequent	May occur, often as onset of severe withdrawal	Convulsions common
Age	Under 35	Age 35-45 Must carefully monitor	Often over age 45 Over age 55
History of DTs	Usually none	Usually none	Has at least one prior occurrence
Last drink	Approx. 12 hours	Approx. 8 hours	Approx 4 hours
Daily consumption (24-hour period)	Less than 1 pint	Over a pint but less than a fifth	Consistently consumes over a fifth

Antabuse®

Most every phase of alcoholism treatment has some controversy attached to it of a pro/con nature. Antabuse is another such area that has been controversial and over which clinicians can argue for hours on end.

Antabuse is a chemical agent that will cause a reaction when mixed with alcohol-containing substances. The chemical name for Antabuse is disulfiram, which is diagrammed in Table 5-II.

Antabuse is a tablet white to off-white and is nearly tasteless. This substance is practically insoluble in water (0.02 g/100ml). The substance is soluble in alcohol, ether, acetone, benzene and

Table 5-II

CHEMICAL FORMULA FOR DISULFIRAM

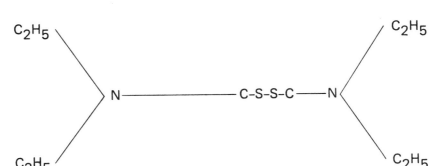

chloroform. Its solubility in alcohol is 3.82 g/100ml and in ether 7.14 g/100 ml.

The ethical considerations for recommending Antabuse therapy require the same thought as any other medication regimen. This point is most important, because Antabuse is a medication regimen just like antibiotics are useful with streptococcal infections. All other objections made about Antabuse somehow obliterate this point. Antabuse is no more intended to be taken for life than is penicillin. Somehow, programs such as Alcoholics Anonymous have members who teach Antabuse is a crutch to keep alcoholics from dealing with their disease.

Some other programs, which have acceptable recovery rates, choose for the patient, in that no patient in their programs is permitted to take Antabuse. The recovery rate cited by these programs is based on the individual's status after one year and almost always include one to three relapses of one day or longer.

Philosophically, each agency must decide if the therapists are to choose for the patient whether Antabuse will or won't be prescribed for some or all of the alcoholics under treatment. While it is doubtful an agency should make such decisions for the clientele without consulting these clients in treatment, many agencies and programs do make such decisions.

Those agencies that make Antabuse available for their clients are responsible to share the risk/benefit factors in detail and obtain an informed consent.

Some of the pros for the Antabuse argument include:

1. It is but a tool that can daily reinforce the initial decision not to drink alcoholic beverages for that day.

2. Antabuse puts precious moments between the urge to drink and when the individual can actually take a drink safely. This stops pressure situations from controlling the individual and gives logic an opportunity to rule.

3. Antabuse offers the individual an opportunity to learn to deal with major psychosocial stressors without drinking. Internal conflicts must now be dealt with instead of being buried in a bottle. Further, individuals facing such stressors benefit tremendously from group therapy (even in an aftercare setting) as they seek to learn to deal with situations never before resolved.

4. The so-called fail-safe period of anywhere from twenty-four hours to fourteen days, depending on the individual, provides the individual an opportunity to ask for help not to drink.

5. Renewed self-confidence flows from the individual because of his/her growth during the period of treatment. The healthy attitude for the individual is, "This will help me through today while my initial recovery is progressing. I will soon be far enough in recovery to not need this medication to assist me."

6. Antabuse, however, also has a frightening list of cons as well. These points are the reason many therapists consider Antabuse too much of a risk to consider using for many patients.

This is a drug/medication. This means that reactions can occur from using other medications, food, and other substances, including cologne. Table 5–III shows the possible reaction to this medication when mixed with alcohol.

Most treating professionals know at least one or two individuals who brag they have taken Antabuse and drank without experiencing these reactions. This is unlikely. Also, all treating professionals know clients who have spit out their Antabuse, put it under their tongue or vomited it up after leaving the nurses station so they can drink when desired. This is unfortunate, yet profes-

Table 5-III

ANTABUSE REACTIONS WITH ALCOHOL

Alcohol Only	Blood Alcohol Level (50mg/100 ml) Release of inhibitions Some loss of judgment	Blood Alcohol Level (100-400mg/ml) Ataxia, combativeness, loss of coordination, loss of all reasoning skills, coma	Blood Alcohol Level (500-800mg/100ml) Death (depresses vital respiratory centers in the brain)
Combination Alcohol/ Antabuse	Blood Alcohol Level (5-10mg/100 ml) Mild reactions (rash, flush, nausea, dizziness) in sensitive individuals	Blood Alcohol Level (50mg/100ml) Full symptoms (blurred vision, confusion, throbbing pain in head and neck, vomiting)	Blood Alcohol Level (125-300mg/ml) Unconsciousness, convulsions, heart failure, death, chest palpitations, dypsnea, hypotension, weakness, vertigo, convulsions, myocardial infarction

sionals should not develop treatment approaches for their whole program based on these few individuals. Many sincerely desire the use of Antabuse and will do well while taking the medication. The remainder will drink *regardless* of what is done for them in treatment.

Management of the reaction to Antabuse must be decisive and immediate (see Table 5-IV).

Elderly persons can be treated with Antabuse if they are in otherwise good health. Usually 75 mg to 125 mg is a sufficient dose to prohibit drinking without incurring side effects.

Listed in Table 5-V are many of the types of medications that contain enough alcohol to cause a reaction in a person taking Antabuse. These medications and compounds are listed by brand names. Many family members have unjustly accused loved ones of returning to alcohol because of the disulfiram reactions that may

Table 5-IV

MANAGEMENT OF THE REACTIVE ANTABUSE PATIENT

Mild Reaction	Moderate Reaction	Severe Reaction
Support	Immediate medical attention	Restore blood pressure
Close supervision	Oxygen	Treat shock
Evaluation by a physician	Maintain airway (possible obstruction if vomiting)	Carbogen (95% oxygen & 5% carbon dioxide)
	Determine what and how much alcohol triggered the reaction	Antioxidant
		Vitamin C by IV (1gr/ 500ml dextrose)
		Also: Ephedrine sulphate, antihistamines, potassium (must be monitored in elderly and heart patients)

be present from medications, aftershaves, and colognes, food and other preparations containing alcohol that were used in all innocence and good faith. Another important point is that this highlights the seriousness of over-the-counter medications, as well as the importance of knowing what an individual is actually taking. The prescribing physician, clinic or agency must be thorough in providing this list to clients and their families while the client is taking Antabuse.

Table 5-V

PRODUCTS CONTAINING ALCOHOL THAT SHOULD BE AVOIDED

ANTI-DIARRHEALS (for diarrhea)
Corrective Mixture®
Corrective Mixture® w/paregoric
Dia-Quel™ liquid
Donnagel® suspension
Donnagel®-PG suspension
Infantol® pink liquid
Lomotil® liquid
Mul-Sed® liquid
Pabizol® w/paregoric
Parelixir® liquid
Parepectolin® suspension
Quintess® suspension

COLD/ALLERGY
Benadryl® elixir
Clistin® elixir
Copavin® compound elixir
CoTylenol® liquid
Demazin® syrup
Dimetane® elixir
Dimetapp® elixir
Fedahist® syrup
Histadyl® syrup
Neo-Synephrine® elixir
Novafed® liquid
Novafed® A liquid
Novahistine® elixir
Ornacol® liquid
Partapp® elixir
Periactin® syrup
Phenergan® syrup
Phenergan® syrup fortis
Poly-Histine® elixir
Propadrine® elixir
Pyribenzamine® elixir
Rohydra® elixir
SK-Diphenhydramine™
Temaril® syrup
Ventilade® syrup

COUGH PREPARATIONS
Actol® expectorant syrup

Acutuss® expectorant w/codeine
Adatuss® cough syrup
Alamine® expectorant
Alamine® liquid
Alamine® C liquid
Ambenyl® expectorant
Anatuss® syrup
Axon® children's cough medicine
Bax® expectorant
Benylin® cough syrup
Breacol®
Broncho-Tussin®
Calcidrine® syrup
Cerose® compound
Cerose DM® expectorant
Cetro Cirose® liquid
Cheracol® syrup
Cheracol® D Cough Syrup
Chlor-Trimeton® expectorant w/codeine
Cidicol® cough formula liquid
Citra® syrup
Citra® forte syrup
Codimal® DH syrup
Codimal® DM syrup
Codimal® PH liquid
Coldene® adult cough formula
Coldene® cough formula (children)
Colrex® compound elixir
Colrex® expectorant
Colrex® syrup
Conar® expectorant
Conar® suspension
Consotuss® antitussive syrup
Coricidin® cough formula syrup
Coryban® D cough syrup
Cosanyl® cough syrup
Cosanyl® DM cough syrup
Cotussis® cough syrup
Creomulsion®
Creo-Terpin®
Dilaudid® cough syrup
Dilocol® syrup
Dimetane® expectorant

Dimetane® expectorant DC
Dimocol® liquid
Diphenhydramine® HCI expectorant
DM®-4 children's cough control
DM®-8 syrup
DM® plus cough syrup
Dorcol® pediatric cough syrup
Dristan® liquid
Entex® liquid
Ephed-Organidin® elixir
Ephedrol® w/codeine liquid
Expectran® DM syrup
FL Tussex® cough syrup
Formula 44D®
2/G® liquid
2/G-DM® liquid
GG-Cen® syrup
GG-Tussin® syrup
Guaiatussin® syrup
Hall's® cough syrup
Histadyl® E.C. syrup
Histavite-D® syrup
Hycotuss® expectorant
Kiddie® cough syrup
Kiddies® pediatric syrup
Mallergan® expectorant w/codeine
Mallergan® VC expectorant w/codeine
Marhist® expectorant
Mercodol® w/decapryn syrup
Minituss® cough syrup
Nilcol® elixir
Noratussin® syrup
Norisodrine® w/calcium iodide syrup
Novahistine® DH liquid
Novahistine® DMX liquid
Novahistine® elixir
Novahistine® expectorant
Nyquil®
Organidin® elixir
Organphen® elixir
Ornacol® liquid
PBZ® expectorant w/codeine and ephedrine
PBZ® expectorant w/ephedrine
Pediacof® cough syrup
Pedituss® liquid
Penetro® syrup
Pertussin® 8-hour liquid
Pertussin® wild berry liquid

Phenacol®-DM syrup
Phenergan® expectorant w/codeine
Phenergan® expectorant pediatric w/dextromethorphan
Phenergan® expectorant plain
Phenergan® VC expectorant w/codeine
Phenergan® VC expectorant plain
Pineutuss-DM® syrup
P-M-Z® HCI expectorant w/codeine
P-M-Z® HCI expectorant plain
Polaramine® expectorant
Promethazine® HCI expectorant w/codeine
Promethazine® HCI expectorant plain
Promethazine® VC expectorant w/codeine
Promex® liquid
Prunicodeine® liquid
Pyraldine® no. 2
Pyraldine® pediatric syrup
Quelidrine® syrup
Quiet-Nite® syrup
Rem® syrup
Rhinex® DM cough syrup
Robitussin® A-C liquid
Robitussin-CF® liquid
Robitussin-DM® syrup
Robitussin-PE® syrup
Robitussin® syrup
Rola-Methazine® decongestant w/codeine
Rola-Methazine® decongestant expectorant plain
Rola-Methazine® expectorant w/codeine
Role-Methazine® expectorant pediatric
Romilar® CF syrup
Romilar® III syrup
Rondec-DM™ drops
Rondec-DM™ syrup
Ryna-Tussadine® expectorant liquid
St. Joseph® cough syrup for children
Special Cough Formula Liquid®
Terpin Hydrate® w/codeine elixir
Terpin Hydrate® w/dextromethorphan hydrobromide elixir
Terpin Hydrate® elixir
Toclonol® w/codeine
Toclonol® expectorant
Tolu-Sed® syrup
Tonecol® syrup
Triaminic® expectorant

Triaminic® expectorant w/codeine
Triaminic® expectorant DH
Trind-DM® syrup
Trind® syrup
Troutman's® syrup
Tuspect® liquid
Tusquelin® syrup
Tussagesic® suspension
Tussar-2® cough syrup
Tussar-SF® cough syrup
Tussend® expectorant
Tussend® liquid
Tussi-Organidin DM™ expectorant
Tussi-Organidin™ expectorant
Tuss-Ornade® liquid
Ulo® syrup
Valdrene® expectorant
Vick's® cough syrup

DENTAL PRODUCTS

Cold Sore/Toothache
Cold Sore Lotion®
Dalidyne® lotion
Dentocaine® (adult)
Dentocaine® (mild)
Dr. Hands® teething gel
Dr. Hands® teething lotion
Jiffy®
Numzit®
Rexall Cold Sore Lotion®
Toothache Drops®

Mouthwash/Gargle
Astring-O-Sol®
Betadine®
Cepacol®
Colgate-100®
Isodine® gargle
Larylgan® throat spray
Lavoris®
Listerine®
Micrin Plus® gargle and rinse
Odara®
Oral Pentacresol®
Scope®

HEMATINICS (for iron deficiency anemia)
Feosol® elixir
Fer-In-Sol® drops

Gerin-In-Sol® syrup
Fetinic-MW® elixir
Fumaral® elixir
Gergon® elixir
Hytinic® elixir
I.L.X.® elixir
Incremin® w/iron syrup
Jeculin® tonic
Li-Betaron® elixir
Mol-Iron® liquid
Neovis® liquid
Niferex® elixir
Nu-Iron® elixir
Pedicran® w/iron liquid
Secran/Fe® elixir
Sorbitinic® liquid

LAXATIVES
Colace® liquid
Cologel® liquid
Doxinate® 5% solution
Dr. Caldwell's Senna Laxative®
Modane® liquid
X-Prep® liquid

VITAMINS/MINERALS (tonics)
Aquasol® E drops
Aquasol® E elixir
Belap® elixir
Belivron® tonic elixir
Beplete® elixir
Betalin® complex elixir
Betalin® S elixir
Bewon® elixir
Bexel® elixir vitamin and iron tonic
Ce-Vi-Sol® drops
Cofron® elixir w/vitamin B_{12}
Crystivite® liquid
Elde-tonic®
Eldiatric® F.S. liquid
Feosol® elixir
Fergon® elixir
Fer-In-Sol® syrup
Ferisorb® liquid
Ganatrex® elixir
Geralix® liquid
Geriplex-FS® liquid
Gerix® elixir
Gerizyme® liquid
Gerizyme® solution

Geroniazol® elixir
Gevrabon® liquid
Gevral® protein powder
Hepp-Iron® elixir w/vitamin B
Homicebrin® liquid
Hytinic® elixir
Iberet® oral solution
Iberet®-500 oral solution
I.L.X.® elixir
Incremin® w/iron syrup
Jeculin® tonic
Lanoplex® elixir
Mol-Iron® liquid
Nicocap® liquid
Nocotinex® elixir
Niferex® elixir
Nu-Iron® elixir
Pedicran® liquid
Poly-Vi-Sol® liquid
Rubraton® elixir
Secran®
Secran® FE elixir
Sorbitinic® liquid
Taka-Combex® elixir
Vi-Daylin® drops
Vi-Daylin® liquid
Vi-Gerol® elixir
Zentron® liquid
Zymalixir® syrup
Zymasyrup®
Zymatinic® drops

PREPARATIONS FOR EXTERNAL APPLICATION

Alkolove® gel
Benzoin® compound tincture
Block Out®
Camphor Spirit®
Chloroform Liniment®
Desenex® solution
Drest Spray®
Feminique®
Green Soap Tincture®
NP-27® liquid
PreSun®
Rhulispray®
Sebucare®
Swim-Ear®

ANTI-ASTHMATIC (for bronchial asthma)

Aerolate® elixir
Asbron® elixir

Asbron G® elixir
Asma® syrup
Ayr® liquid
Broncholate® elixir
Brondecon® elixir
Bronkodyl® elixir
Bronkolixir®
Choledyl® elixir
Co-Xan® elixir
Decadron® elixir
Dilor® elixir
Elixodyne® elixir
Elixophyllin® elixir
Elixophyllin-Kl® elixir
Embron® syrup
Ephedrine® sulfate syrup
G-Bron® elixir
Glynazan® elixir
Isuprel® compound elixir
Lanophyllin® elixir
Lixaminol AT® liquid
Lixaminol® elixir
Lufyllin® elixir
Lufyllin® EPG elixir
Lufyllin® GG elixir
Maras® DF syrup
Marax® syrup
Mini-Lix® elixir
Mudrane® GG elixir
Neothylline® elixir
Neothylline®-G elixir
Norisodrine® w/calcium iodide syrup
Panophylline® forte elixir
Quibron® elixir
Quibron® plus elixir
Synophylate® elixir
Synophylate®-GG syrup
Tedral® elixir
Tega-Bron® elixir
Theofort elixir
Theo-Guaia® liquid
Theokin® elixir
Theo-lix® elixir
Theolixir®
Theolline®
Theo-Organidin® elixir
Theon® elixir
Theophyl®-225 elixir
Theophylline® elixir
Theo-11® elixir
Theospan® syrup
TSG-Kl® elixir

Chapter 6

MENTAL HEALTH/PSYCHOTHERAPY

Psychotherapy

MANY mental health centers have not realized how successful short term psychotherapy can be with the elderly. This pessimism is not justified. Some of the pessimism regarding psychotherapy and the aged can be traced to the stereotype of all senior citizens as being senile. Thus, medical intervention is not sought to isolate the cause of the confusion, forgetfullness, paranoid reactions, hypochrondriasis, situational disturbances, and anxiety.

The expectations of many senior citizens entering therapy are more realistic than their younger counterparts. They do not expect to have a miracle performed for them. Because many see their life span as limited, they often resolve issues much more quickly. The elderly psychotherapy client tends to savour even a little progress as satisfying and worthwhile. As an understanding is made regarding positive mental health changes, the stigma about asking for help is removed. People who seek mental health services are no longer labeled as crazy.

Many elderly persons are entering a therapeutic relationship simply to improve the quality of their life. For clinics offering socialization groups and activities, those clients are often only lonely. Most of the behavioral and personality-related causes of confusion, loneliness, depression, and suicidal ideation are most amenable to psychotherapy in this age-group.

The reasons for this myth continuing to be believed are two-fold. First, successful adaptation for the elderly is dependent on a

90

multiplicity of factors. Some of these are the person's health, income, standard of living, living arrangements, social contacts, transportation, family, and degree of loss. Secondly, successful adaptation in younger years does not guarantee being able to function in the elderly years.

The key is often the degree of loss, which is often cumulative in the elderly. The following Cumulative Loss Questionnaire shown in Figure 6-1 shows many of the losses to which the individual is asked to adapt and cope.

CUMULATIVE LOSS QUESTIONNAIRE©

CATEGORY	YEAR OF LOSS	RESPONSE
DEATH Spouse Child Grandchild Sibling Friends		
HEALTH Chronic Pain Acute Illness Alcoholism Prescription Drug Misuse Over the Counter Medication Misuse		
MENTAL HEALTH Personal Confrontation with Mortality Chronic Pain Significant Illness of Spouse Less Sexual Satisfaction Loss of Opportunity to Achieve Life Goals		
PHYSICAL CHANGE Loss of Reserve Capacity Sensory Loss - Vision Sensory Loss - Hearing Slowing of Responsiveness		
RETIREMENT Decline of Income Change of Life Roles Stress on Marriage Change of Family Home		
OTHER LOSSES Loss of Mobility Loss of Independence Institutionalization Inflation Disengagement Crime Victim Changing Physical Appearance		

Figure 6-1. This questionnaire can enable the clinician to better understand the client's losses, sequence, and how the client copes.

Several factors influence the magnitude of losses and the individual's response to the loss. The first factor is the frequency of loss. Losses occurring closely together tend to become synergistic (i.e. the impact of the loss is geometrically greater than the sum of the loss). When the deaths of several significant people occur within a one- or two-year span, then the losses become unbearable. The second factor is the individual's established pattern for dealing with stress and loss. Individuals with a life pattern of coping with stress successfully are often most able to cope with a major loss in late life. However, losses are cumulative. Individuals each have a breaking point in their coping skills.

Therapists need to ask clients this question, "What event or combination of life circumstances would cause you to consider taking your life?" If clients deal with this beforehand, then the chances for a suicidal response decrease. Even the strongest character can be challenged to the breaking point. "Survivors" are particularly at-risk clients in this process. How long can anyone take continuing loss without need of help?

Mrs. J was sixty-nine years old when she first sought mental health assistance. She was brought to the agency by one of her two sisters who had noticed suicidal ideation. Mrs. J was blind in both eyes. She had suffered a degenerating eye disease at age thirty and was blind by age thirty-three. She successfully completed blind school training and was fluent in the use of Braille. She was employed by the Library for the Blind. One of her great joys was reading books onto cassette tapes to enable others to enjoy them. She was married twice and widowed both times. She described prolonged depression, but stated that she overcame this by continuing to work. Her one child did all she could, but lived out of state and was the mother of two also. Retirement was forced on her and again she coped, although depressed. She did not become suicidal until a sudden hearing loss. She was devastated by so cruel a loss as her hearing upon which she so heavily depended.

This kind of tragic case is not uncommon among the elderly. Therapy with such a case is indeed difficult and the prognosis is poor. The therapist, in a case such as the above, must utilize strengths, rebuild social support and give considerable support.

Secondly, therapeutic techniques require that the traditional psychotherapeutic techniques be modified. Ineffective techniques with the elderly include psychoanalytic style approaches.

The effective gerontologist is one who understands some of the changes associated with the elderly. These include:

1. *Fatigability:* The elderly person will tend to tire more quickly, making longer sessions inadvisable.
2. *Hearing Loss:* All elderly persons experience some degree of hearing loss so that voice levels must be adjusted accordingly.
3. *Chronic Pain:* Clients with arthritis, injury and some depressive syndromes are unable to sit and are unable to concentrate over a few minutes. The therapist must be amenable to changing chairs, standing and even breaks in the middle of the therapy session.
4. *Transportation Difficulty:* The therapist must be flexible in appointment times when the patient is dependent on others for transportation to and from appointments.
5. *Financial Limitations:* At the present, Medicare pays only $250/year for outpatient psychotherapy. Since many elderly persons are living on fixed incomes, long-term therapy costs are prohibitive.
6. *Intellectual Functioning:* Less than 10 percent of all elderly clients have any limitation to intellectual functioning. Thus, the client is probably not limited in understanding.

The effective therapist will exhibit several qualities that will facilitate improvement in the elderly client:

1. *Dynamic:* The therapist must be active, involved and verbal in sessions. Although many therapists loathe the role of advice giver, sometimes clients require the therapist's viewpoint be given. As long as the clients understand the decision rests on them, this is seldom problematic.
2. *Warmth:* This population requires what Carl Rogers called "empathic understanding." The therapist must exhibit concern, caring, and compassion in the relationship.

3. *Informal Setting:* Experience indicates that the more informal the approach to therapy, the more productive the sessions.

4. *Limited Scope of Therapy:* Often the individual requires assistance/therapy with one or two concerns. The goals tend to be limited and quite specific.

5. *Supportive Therapy:* Many of the difficulties facing senior citizens simply cannot be "fixed." The death of a loved one or friend, the lack of income, caring for a disabled relative, Alzheimer's disease, and chronic health problems simply have no therapeutic remedy. Thus, support, grief therapy and "a shoulder to cry on" are essential.

6. *Advocacy:* The therapist must be a referral source for clients and should be able to identify the physicians, attorneys, psychiatrists, pharmacists and other professionals who are knowledgeable of the elderly and willing to accept them for assistance. Occasionally, intervention with other social service systems on behalf of the client is advisable and necessary.

7. *Accurate Diagnosis:* Organic brain syndrome is not the major mental health concern of the elderly. *Depression* and *alcoholism* are competing for the number one and two positions of frequency. Misdiagnosis dooms therapy before it begins. If more than 10 percent of all elderly patients in any setting are diagnosed organic brain syndrome, then aggressive review of the reason and appropriate staff training need to occur.

Diagnostic Issues

Emotional difficulties should not be treated symptomatically. Various professionals must diagnose cause of the symptoms, then refer them for treatment by a therapist. By treating symptoms, the physician often medicates the spouse of an alcoholic, thus enabling the *family* disease and dysfunction to continue, or gives a prescription for pills to the chemically dependent person. Neither of these is a therapeutically or medically sound procedure. All minor/major tranquilizers should be prescribed by competent psychiatric personnel *after thorough* assessment.

"I'm nervous all the time. I haven't slept a night for several weeks. The lump in my stomach keeps my food from settling." Thus, the doctor referred this sixty-nine-year-old person to the mental health clinic for evaluation/treatment when medical tests revealed no reason for this difficulty. Clinical assessment revealed that she was the wife and sister of two alcoholics, both of whom she served as a caretaker and neither of whom she helped.

Mrs. X, forty-seven years old, complained of tension headaches. She was convinced they were of a cause to "make me crazy." She had been to a medical doctor, but only for a "physical." She presented herself to the clinic "for anything to help the pain." When asked about her marriage, she stated, "we get along like most people, we argue some." Clinical assessment revealed that the arguments were physical fights following her husband's night of drinking, which had progressed from "once every few months" to every weekend. These fights were ending with physical abuse to her person.

Clinical assessment must include careful questioning as to drinking history. The percentage of Americans who abstain totally from the beverage alcohol is approximately 15 percent. Thus, assume that the person drinks and ask several direct questions regarding frequency/amount consumed. The majority of clients will not be offended by the question and will answer directly and simply. The more someone qualifies or indicates outrage at the question, the closer the clinician needs to look at the issue.

As discussed earlier, the clinician must be comfortable diagnosing alcoholism as a primary disease, and all clinicians must be made aware of their own use of alcohol. Alcoholism is the problem whether diagnosed or not. Treatment is a sham if the real problem isn't even diagnosed.

Further, as physicians are undertrained to deal with alcoholism, so also are social workers, counselors, gerontologists, psychologists and medication clinic personnel. However, the mental health agencies must train their staff to recognize alcoholism and to accept this as a course of therapy. The agency is negligent in prescribing any medication for a patient without assessing alcohol intake.

Moreover, much could be said about the DSM III guidelines on alcohol-related diagnoses and the sister codes, ICD 9-CM. Not one code exists to facilitate alcoholism treatment of the family as the primary focus of dysfunction. Instead, the significant others end up with such non-useful diagnosis as "unspecified personality disorder." Clinicians will not diagnose these disorders, and third-party payments will not be received until such time as a diagnostic code *exists* for the dysfunction. The DSM III was revised without such a code, which insures continuing dysfunction for forty million Americans (each of the ten million alcoholics adversely affect four other persons around them). This is a critical and costly oversight by those counted upon to guide the profession.

Medication Issues

Another primary concern for professionals treating alcoholism and coalcoholism in a mental health setting is one of prescribing medication to alleviate emotional difficulties. The risk of prescribing medication for the alcoholic is well documented. However, it is not as well documented for the coalcoholic, who is often the one who will come into treatment in the mental health setting for a nervous condition.

Mrs. K was such an individual. She arrived on advice from her doctor swearing she had cancer of the colon; minimally an ulcer. A carefully detained history and well-asked questions by the interviewer produced the classic coalcoholic (living with an alcoholic husband and mimicking his behavior). She demanded that in order to come back to treatment that she be given something to alleviate this stress. The professional declined, informing her that it was neither prudent nor helpful for her to become dependent on mood-altering medications anymore than it is prudent for her husband to be addicted to alcohol. She was encouraged to come in for outpatient therapy two times a week for the first three weeks, then once a week thereafter on a long-range basis.

She did agree and was given literature to review. It was not until the second month of treatment when she had developed some inner resources of her own that an appointment was scheduled for her to see the psychiatrist. At that time, she was put on a very mild stomach relaxer to help her digestion during times of upset.

When alcoholism or any other chemical abuse is present in a household, much careful thought must be given to whether or not to introduce another chemical into that family system. Accidental overdose, suicide and numerous other possibilities that often hamper getting the alcoholic into treatment can occur if it is the coalcoholic for whom the medication is prescribed. Also, when treating the coalcoholic, it is important to recognize that very often that person is consuming a fair amount of alcohol themselves; often under the guise that if they drink with the other alcoholic, this person will be safer and they will know where the alcoholic is.

Medication should only be prescribed a coalcoholic after the therapist has seen this person a number of times and knows within reasonable probability that alcohol will not be mixed with the medication setting up an accidental overdose or death. When treating the elderly couple alcoholic/coalcoholic situation, this question becomes extremely important. Profound health problems occur much more often for the coalcoholic of an elderly age as a result of the stress that the person endures, particularly if the alcoholic is a phase-of-life addicted drinker. Thus, careful insight must be given to the type of medication prescribed and how that medication interacts with other medications that the person may be on as a result of failing health.

Always keep in mind that the individual's liver and excretory systems slow down with age; so, the medication will not be excreted as rapidly from the system as it is in the younger counterpart. A psychotropic medication on top of drugs such as Inderal®, Indocin®, Digoxin® or similar medications can have a profoundly serious impact. Further, tricyclic anti-depressive medications, which are often called for from the coalcoholic elderly, may result in a drug overdose of a different nature because of the mixture of medications that should not be mixed.

It is important to remember that in a society where people want to take a pill and feel better, it is hard to explain sometimes to these individuals that giving them this medication can, in fact, cause them serious harm as opposed to alleviating the difficulty that brought them in for treatment. Often, the psychiatrists in the mental health setting are not familiar enough with these mixtures of drugs and the potential effect. It is incumbent upon the therapists to share with them so that the elderly are not set up in a very dangerous situation.

It is obligatory that the mental health professional monitor the mixture of drugs rather than the private physician, presuming that the mental health professionals are the experts in the psychotropic field, on those medications prescribed, and with what they can and cannot be mixed. Since elderly persons often do not know to ask those questions, the mental health professional is in every sense ethically and professionally bound to protect the interest of the client.

Further, since most of the elderly do not have a great deal of knowledge of medicines and their interactions in the system and are not likely to retain the information given verbally, it behooves the individual providing the treatment to give this information on the medication (and the side effects and the food and medicines that should be avoided) to the elderly individuals in writing. Thus, the person will have an immediate paper in hand to refer to if in doubt.

The issue of prescribing psychotropic medication for the alcoholic becomes even more of a difficult question. Though the goal of every treatment approach known in the field is that the person will not return to drinking once treatment is completed, a significant question to be dealt with is: Can you really take a chance on this individual not returning to drinking? For the elderly alcoholic, there are some key indicators; if the person still has a child or children in the area, still has his or her wife/husband, has some hobbies that are feasible to return to, and if it is not extremely difficult to get help, then the chance is very good that the person will not return to drinking. However, if those things are absent and the therapist is attempting to rebuild the social structure, relapse is almost always a cetainty at some point in the road.

Relapse, if on psychotropic medication, sets up an immediate life-threatening situation. Thus, it may be very important to either not prescribe the medication or to prescribe it in such low dosages that the person is not likely to kill him/herself if he/she does relapse. Further, frequent clinic visits for medication are desirable so that the medication is not on hand if relapse occurs. This approach might raise eyebrows in terms of whether or not the therapist is actually setting up relapse by not prescribing the medication; however, in an advocacy role (which therapists are), these factors must be taken into account when prescribing chemicals.

Another factor to be weighed in the prescription dilemmas is whether or not you want to risk having the person depend on yet another chemical to control moods and to alleviate stress and difficulty. Often, it is preferable to keep the individual off all things, including over-the-counter medications, so that the person learns to deal with life without a chemical additive to support him or her. Although much has been written about this dilemma, and many treatment programs have the philosophy about this, it is not always the same in every case and, regardless of the policy plausibility, must be maintained also. A good case example follows:

Mr. M was seen in an emergency room evaluation, had returned to drinking and had his prescription in his pocket — two bottles of the same medication. The stressor in his returning to drink was the fact that his wife had been given ten days to live, seven days prior to being evaluated. The client was understandably under enough stress that some form of medication relief was necessary, or the person would drink to find that relief. He was subsequently hospitalized on an inpatient unit, and a social worker accompanied him on his last visit to see his wife and throughout her dying process.

Although such a case may seem rare, incidents such as these are very prevalent among the elderly, especially on oncology units. Thus, we must be alerted to when the person is in such severe distress that some form of relief is not only desirable but essential. Again, such a plan of action must be carefully monitored because in times of stress, such as the death of a spouse or a child, or forced retirement after many years of service, the individual who has been sober for a good many years may very easily return to the bottle for relief.

Self-Love

The issue of ego strength, self-worth, or self-esteem is the most difficult for mental health persons to rebuild. All chemically dependent persons must be treated for lack of self-esteem. Daniel Anderson (Hazelden, 1976) states, "Self-esteem is made up of at least three components: a sense of being effective, a sense of worthiness, and a sense of immortality."

The alcoholic and coalcoholic both require therapy in these three spheres. Often, the marriage has deteriorated to the point that each can only tell the therapist and each other what is wrong with their spouse. These feelings and negative attitudes are generalized back throughout the marriage. The desperate state of unhappiness is evident in the spouse's opinions of self and the spouse.

Sobriety will never result until the self-love or self-esteem is rebuilt. Often, the therapist must probe and teach to get the couple to share one positive quality about the other. The individual's thinking must be restructured to the positive realm. This is difficult, indeed, if both spouses are not in therapy.

Once sober, the alcoholic must begin to deal with the shambles that their life is in. The anxiety is heightened by the sense that somehow failure will result regardless of the effort the individual makes. Perhaps this is the one factor that is most influencing of the relapse potential. The more someone has tried to quit on their own and failed, the greater the anxiety.

Alcoholics Anonymous and Treatment Program Alumni Associations are the most effective in combatting this kind of anxiety. The power to overcome is obvious when those who have shared with those who are struggling. Many times these volunteers can best answer the "how" questions. Theory and education alone will not produce sobriety and family recovery. The practical "how to" must also be given.

Another key area to be treated is that of moodiness. Much discussion is given to this in the treatment chapters. However, as is the case with all emotional difficulties, thorough assessment must be done.

Depression

The major mental health problem in elderly alcoholics is depression. Research is still being conducted to determine whether depression triggers alcoholism in phase-of-life drinking. Clinical evidence suggests that depression is closely linked to escalating drinking in this age bracket.

Differentiation must be made between endogenous depression and reactive depressions. Of the two, the reactive depressions are the most dangerous for the alcoholic.

Symptoms of Reactive Depression	*Endogenous Depression*
Anxiety	Excessive sleep
Restlessness	Sad
Insomnia	Hopelessness
Irritable	Decreased sex drive
Fatigue	Withdrawn
Feelings of guilt and anger	Poor appetite
Crying spells	Psychomotor retardation
Expresses helplessness and inadequacy	Suicidal thoughts
Impaired concentration	

Medications are helpful with endogenous depression. The epinephrine levels are increased in the brain and the depressed mood is decreased, thus making therapy beneficial.

Medications are less helpful with reactive depressions. The principle reason is that often the causes of reactive depressions are losses that cannot be replaced. Therefore, medication is not going to help significantly either.

One case is that of an elderly woman whose husband had died two years previously. Due to being prescribed a tranquilizer to ease her grief, she had been sedated against grieving at all. Once the drug was withdrawn, she went into the grief reaction she should have experienced two years earlier. Such a case is not rare. Medications are actually harmful at such a time as this. The normal, human emotion at the death of a spouse is to grieve, especially after good marriages of long duration.

A note of caution, however. The therapist must be sure to understand the client's reaction within the client's values. The therapist's shoulds and values can tremendously hamper therapy if the therapist attributes them wrongly to the client.

Depression is also a normal reaction to loss. Depression becomes of concern when it lasts longer than a month or when consideration of suicide is prevalent. Each transient suicidal ideation is relatively normal. Most people in times of tremendous loss and stress think, "I wish I were dead" or "I just can't face tomorrow." Most persons who experience this are mutually healthy enough to dismiss the thought as extreme. Those who carry the ideation through to a plan need immediate intensive therapy.

The data on the use of tricyclic anti-depressants is not conclusive. However, clinical evidence suggests that these medications may be most beneficial in assisting the alcoholic to even out moods, while striving to build a meaningful sobriety.

Empty Nest Syndrome

That career housewives and mothers experience a tremendous loss when the youngest child leaves home is well accepted. Many of these women in the 40-50-year-old age bracket require assistance in rebuilding a more meaningful life-style.

The phenomenon that has not received much attention is the fathers who experience the same phenomena as the women. These men include those disabled due to war or illness who were primary caretakers of the children during significant phases of child rearing. As role reversals continue, this is going to be more evident as a therapy need.

The other aspect of the empty nest syndrome that has received little attention is the transference from the youngest child to the grandchild or grandchildren. No harm usually comes from such a transference until geographical or other circumstances interfere with these relationships. When treating familial problems, the therapist must be careful to probe exactly how the children left home. Many of the resentments and family strife arise out of the inability for the child to leave home without such an uproar. Many times, the anger is simply an enabling factor to allow the separations. Such cases require a careful combination of confrontation and support.

Such programs as volunteering in a pediatric ward at a hospital, working with scouting programs, foster grandparents, and other opportunities can be utilized when distance prohibits involvement with family. All therapists who work with the elderly need to be familiar with these programs and how to refer to them.

SELECTED READINGS FOR
MENTAL HEALTH PROFESSIONALS

Butler, R.N., and Lewis, M.I.: *Aging and Mental Health, Positive Psycho-Social Approaches.* St. Louis, C. V. Mosby, 1977.
Zarit, S.H.: *Aging and Mental Disorders: Psychological Approaches to Assessment and Treatment.* New York: Free Press, 1980.

Chapter 7

POLY DRUG MISUSE

Statistical Prevalence

A SURVEY of prescription and other over-the-counter medications was conducted with a substantial number of elderly persons. The individuals were simply asked to list all those medications taken within the last thirty days. The results were astounding!

Ninety-five percent of all persons over age 65 failed to list over-the-counter (OTC) medications on the questionnaire even though 67 percent were taking at least one item. When queried, each stated that these medications were not the same as those prescribed by physicians. Further questioning revealed that only 17 percent of the patients were using OTC medications on the advice of physicians, which included aspirin, hemorrhoid preparations, vitamins, muscle relaxers, laxatives and similar medications.

Statistically, persons over age 65 make up about 10 percent of the population but use 25 percent of all prescriptions written by physicians. This means 225 million prescriptions are written for this age group annually. Over 80 percent of the prescriptions are for mood-altering substances, such as sleeping pills, anti-depressants and sedative-hypnotic drugs. Of the remaining 20 percent of medications prescribed, the largest number are for chronic pain and arthritis.

The National Council on Aging estimates that 20 percent of all out-of-pocket health expenses are for drugs.

No one interviewed in any of the surveys were living drug-free lives. This is a reflection of the times in which we live. The mentality that makes prescription drug addiction the elderly's foremost health hazard is influenced by several factors.

First, the prevailing attitude in all age groups is that the office visit to the physician is wasted unless she/he prescribes at least one medication. The diagnosis is no longer significant, only the "cure."

Secondly, patients expect instant relief no matter what the condition under treatment is. To be told that a medicine will take twenty-one days to work (as in the case with most psychotropics) is, as one patient phrased it, "to abandon me to needless suffering." Of course, the patient tolerated her symptoms for almost two years before seeking treatment.

Thirdly, advertisers invariably promise "instant relief" from their OTC substances, thus raising expectations that prescription drugs will exceed these "less important" medications. Much more stringent controls need to be placed on advertising. For example, a current laxative commercial begins by the lady holding a pill in her hand while the voice tells her what all this pill will accomplish. She exclaims, "This little pill does all that!" Thus, several clients have asked the psychiatrist if their "little pill" has enough medication to successfully treat the condition. The size of the pill has nothing at all to do with the effects of the pill. Haldol®, Inderal®, Antivert®, and Nitroglyn® are but a few extremely powerful "little pills."

Fourthly, no individual expects to suffer any amount of discomfort at any time. The unwritten rule is to seek immediate relief by some means as soon as onset occurs. No longer are non-medication means even thought about, much less tried (such as relaxation techniques for stress-related headaches, warm milk for insomnia, and the like). Further compounding this problem is the use of alcoholic beverages for self-medicating anxiety, insomnia and depression to name the major ailments. Clients have also reported drinking themselves into oblivion to escape dealing with chronic pain. The causes of chronic pain include arthritis, pain from old injuries and back ailments. Since depression is a major cause of lower back pain in the elderly, careful diagnosis must be accomplished.

The next danger of even more importance is the practice of prescription swapping that is done among family members and in settings such as retirement communities. The myth is that such swapping is done in ignorance and is careless. Often, this is not the case. Prescription trading is a practice that is here to stay. To tell people not to trade medications is useless. This is true for several reasons:

1. Many persons have become knowledgable of drug trade names and the symptoms corrected by the medication. Thus, they have no qualms about sharing.
2. They are satisfied with the cure they have received so they share with their neighbors who are suffering a similar ill.
3. Some kinds of conditions are common to specific families so that several persons may use the same kind of medication. So, when one member runs out, another will "loan" the extra medications.
4. Prescriptions are expensive. Although the generic drug program has helped, medications are costly. The cost to visit a physician and receive 1-2 medications ranges from $30-$60. Thus, swapping saves money.
5. Medications are quality controlled for freshness so that the prescriptions can be stored for later use.

Some remedial steps to prohibit the practice from reaching tragic proportions are:

1. Physicians to write smaller prescriptions with a refill. Although this approach had drawbacks, this prohibits large numbers of pills from being on hand.
2. Change of law that allows the return of unused medications. Each person can recount drugs that were prescribed and filled and then discontinued because of side effects or symptom change. Thus, whole prescriptions are left sitting.
3. Physicians can use drug company samples for trials of medications prior to writing a prescription. Thus, many problems can be worked out before prescriptions are purchased.
4. Education concerning dangers of medications if used improperly. Also, if symptoms are masked, then proper diagnosis is not possible (as is the case when someone uses another's medications).

5. Pharmacists should be utilized more often to choose appropriate medications and dosages. The pharmacist is the most underutilized health professional.
6. People need to choose one pharmacists and have *all* prescriptions filled at this pharmacy. This allows a knowledgable health professional to assist in medications.
7. Physicians need to be more diligent about knowing exactly what other doctors are prescribing the patient. Many medications are highly dangerous if taken in combination. The responsibility is on the physician to check on this prior to prescribing anything.

Patterns of Dependence

Prescription Use

Surveys have consistently found that over one-third of those who use prescription drugs use at least two prescriptions concurrently. Those who have responded in such surveys are often women who report at least one major health condition.

The leading causes of reported ill health are cardiovascular, hypertension, arthritis and mental health difficulties (e.g. insomnia, depression, anxiety and grief).

Studies have consistently found that anywhere from 40 percent to 70 percent of the persons over age 65 report needing their medication to carry out their daily activities. Almost without exception, the persons knew what their medications were and the action the medications had in their body.

Psychotropic drugs are among the highest number of prescriptions written and are by far the most dangerous when mixed with alcohol. These may also be the easiest to become dependent upon because of their mood-stabilizing effect. The debate has been going on for many years about whether these dependencies are physiological or psychological in nature. The argument has somehow exempted anyone from treating the problem while the issue is debated. Based on statistical data, the professional can assume that it is both!

Every alcohol program can tell stories of persons who were detoxified and placed in treatment, only to be returned to the detox unit in a few days. The problem? Valium®, Librium®, Dalmane®, and similar kinds of prescriptions, taken over time, had been discontinued. The individual was now in withdrawal once more.

Every medication taken to have a certain action also causes an opposite reaction. A sleeping medication that calms and sedates will cause mild agitation three to four hours later. This is why many persons report waking after this period of time and being unable to fall back asleep.

Antibiotics are one of the most medically revolutionary discoveries of all time. This class of drugs is also frequently abused. Many takers do not realize that an antibiotic kills *all* the bacteria in a person's body, the good (urinary tract, digestive tract) and the bad (whatever the infection is). Thus, side effects are often a secondary infection.

The other frequent medication is overdose, which occurs in this age bracket in one of three ways:

1. Willful overdose that occurs when someone decides upon this as a means to commit suicide.
2. The erroneous idea that taking an extra dose will work twice as fast. Thus, the person often takes too much and incurs the discomfort of this practice.
3. Physicians *frequently* give the elderly too high a dose of medication. As a rule, a dose of half to two-thirds the amount is therapeutic for someone over age 70, if in good health, and age 60 if in poor health.

Polyannie demonstrates the frequent observable signs of over-medication (both psychotropic and medication use for physical illness).

Figure 7-1 shows the shuffling gait. This needs to be evaluated with common sense. If the person has always shuffled along, this may be normal. However, if last week the person was walking upright and freely and this week is shuffling, then the cause is not old age.

Figure 7-2 demonstrates akathisia, or difficulty in sitting still. Tremors may be evident. This is particularly important to evaluate if the client is taking one of the anti-depressant medications.

Figure 7-2 demonstrates Polyannie suffering from dystonia, which is the back arching, neck drawing up and the upward gaze! This is a side effect commonly attributed to Haldo and similar medications. This symptom, also referred to as EPS (extrapyramidal stimulation) may well need counter-medication.

Figure 7-1 shows Polyandy with a masked, glazed-over expression. This is a common symptom when the client is taking several medications at one time. When coupled with confusion, the first diagnostic probe needs to be the amount of medications consumed. This symptom can also occur when alcohol is mixed with anti-pain or anti-anxiety medications. Figure 7-1 also demonstrates the involuntary salivations that at times occur.

Again, diagnoses must be swift and complete. Elderly persons who suffer strokes may suddenly manifest a shuffling gait, involuntary salivation and a masked expression. Immediate medical help is required at any manifestation of such symptoms.

Over-the-Counter Medications

More elderly persons use OTC medications daily than consume prescription drugs. One study reports the difference as 69 percent using OTC while 55.4 percent used prescription medications (Guttman).

The OTC preparations most commonly being used by the elderly include internal analgesics, laxatives, vitamins and some of the antihistamine and cold remedies.

The other surprising statistical finding is that only one-sixth of all persons who use OTC medications report consulting their physician first.

In conclusion, one point must be considered. Poly drug use is common, safe and necessary. Many people are alive today because of a carefully prescribed combination of life-sustaining drugs. However, poly drug *misuse* is also common. This is dangerous and can bring about death or incapacitation. This is the class of misuse that is frequently fatal if mixed with alcohol. The difference is great between poly drug use and poly drug abuse.

POLYANDY EXHIBITS MAJOR SYMPTOMS OF POLY-DRUG MISUSE

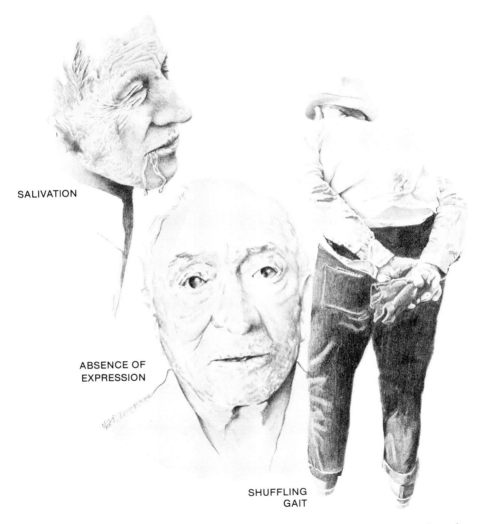

SALIVATION

ABSENCE OF
EXPRESSION

SHUFFLING
GAIT

Figure 7-1. *Right,* The client with a shuffling gait is not exhibiting a sign of old age. Rather, prescription drug overuse and/or alcohol use should be suspected. *Center,* The masked face and absence of expression can be from several causes. Prescription use must be evaluated. *Left,* Uncontrolled salivation has two main causes — prescription overuse and stroke.

POLYANNIE EXHIBITS SYMPTOMS OF POLY-DRUG MISUSE

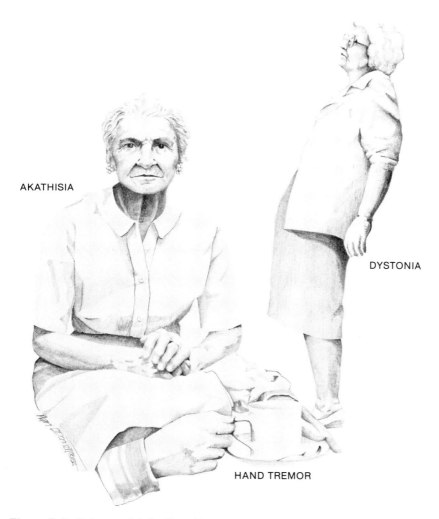

AKATHISIA

DYSTONIA

HAND TREMOR

Figure 7-2. *Below and left,* The client with restlessness, impaired concentration, fine body tremor and shaking hands may well be an overdose victim of medication. *Right,* Unlike other symptoms with possible other causes, this condition *is* from medication overdose. Often, as is the case with psychotropic medications, the corrective action is to countermedicate.

Chapter 8

THE ELDERLY ALCOHOLIC AS A UNIQUE TREATMENT POPULATION

Background and Statistical Information

STATISTICALLY, there are approximately 4 million alcoholics age 60 and over in the United States today. As the number of Americans reaching this age group increases, so will the alcoholism rate. Yet only approximately 2 percent of alcoholics in this age bracket are sober. Obviously, treatment programs and outreach programs are not educating and reaching senior citizens who are struggling with alcohol addiction.

A senior citizen in today's culture (someone in their 70s) matured in a generation that saw alcohol linked with every kind of crime and vicious practices of all sorts and lived through Prohibition. This generation more than any other has seen the stigma against men and women who were called weak willed, who were considered immoral, and who were ridiculed as having lost control of their lives. A simple twenty-one or twenty-eight day treatment program will not undo this lifetime of belief of judging and seeing others judged as weak willed and unable to handle life. This person will probably need some intensive individual counseling, literature to read and very often will not accept the disease concept no matter with what sincerity this concept is taught to them. Treatment personnel must be sensitive to this and treat the addiction. Therapy is not a doctrinal issue (i.e. the person must accept the disease concept with sobriety, being the award for belief).

Because of the senior citizen's age, they don't have the ten, fifteen, or twenty years to develop the usual progression that is associated with alcoholism without getting some help. Because of the physiological changes that the body undergoes naturally, the body is less able to cope with alcohol abuse. Because nutritional deprivation, organ damage, brain damage, diseases and other physiological consequences of drinking are apt to be severe, the elderly alcoholic often literally dies before ever seeking treatment. Compounding this problem is the fact that today's seventy- and eighty-year-old alcoholics have always considered that illnesses are to be overcome without a physician's help. Even if treatment was considered, most would not know where to turn to receive this desired treatment.

Unfortunately, for these alcoholics, the natural consequences of drinking often take total control of their life before ever seeking some form of treatment to enhance the chances for sobriety. The elderly alcoholic is more apt to drink alone and be isolated in either their own peer group (i.e. a senior citizen's living area) or simply drink in their homes by themselves. This occurs for a couple of reasons:

1. The elderly cannot afford the prices charged at such a gathering as a cocktail lounge, dance, or similar gathering.
2. The elderly alcoholic is more apt to be conscious of public embarrassment and to avoid such risks as being arrested while driving or to be seen staggering in public. Those alcoholics who are arrested or seen in public are signaling the severity of their alcoholism.

The elderly alcoholic is very often apt to develop an intolerance to alcohol. This is due to body organ's decreasing ability to process alcohol and to the often cross-use of prescription drugs. Also, the ratio of body water increases with age. Alcohol is soluble in water but is not soluble in fat, resulting in higher concentration of alcohol in the brain and bloodstream. This problem is even more severe in women than in men. Combined with slower metabolism, this results in a higher concentration of alcohol for a longer period of time. While their younger counterparts metabolize one ounce of alcohol per hour, the elderly alcoholic metabolizes a half ounce to three-fourths of an ounce per hour.

When an alcoholic in this age bracket is brought into the emergency room, very often even the doctor will mistake the staggering, slurring of speech, the incoherence and the confusion as an evidence of senility rather than alcoholism. Often, if the family doctor has been the treating physician of an individual for a long period of time, the physician will admit the elderly alcoholic to a hospital, knowing full well that it is alcoholism for which they are being hospitalized and yet, rather than "embarrass" the individual, will give some other kind of diagnosis to them. Thus, a denial syndrom in society itself keeps the alcoholic out of treatment in this age group.

The elderly alcoholic is very apt to blame his drinking on a somatic complaint such as arthritis or pain associated with some other injury. This phenomenon is as exacerbated by alcohol aggravating chronic health conditions and by the central nervous system's depressive effects of alcohol, which makes the pain more bearable. This pain relief is obtained on a short-term basis, but the condition causing the pain is made worse. As shown in Figure 8-1, the cycle repeats itself with disasterous results.

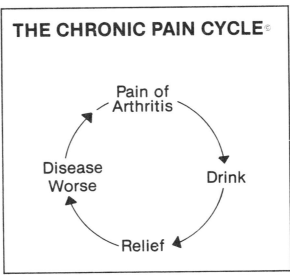

Figure 8-1. Chronic pain relief is one of the major problems that the elderly face, especially if no medical remedy for the cause of the pain can be rendered.

Eventually, the drinker has to come to the point where the pain that they're drinking to escape is less than the pain that is being caused by their drinking. This often is called "hitting bottom" in the AA literature and other treatment literature. The elderly alcoholic more so than probably any other drinker needs that bottom to be raised for them, rather than they being left to hit the bottom.

Often an inability to cope with retirement is a common denominator for senior citizens with drinking problems. Very few men and women actually know what the retirement years are going to bring to their life and often do not plan them with the realistic sense of what this role holds for them. The overwhelming majority of the senior citizens who are now alcoholics in this culture drink minimum amounts of alcohol socially prior to retirement. The majority of alcoholics in this age group have increased dramatically their alcohol consumption since their retirement. Alcoholics in this age bracket are very apt to drink to relieve tension and the stresses brought on by the retirement process. This is not denial. Alcoholics over sixty are much more influenced by events they were formerly able to manage than their counterparts.

As the individual age increases, environmental manipulation must be a major focus of treatment; to the extent environmental factors can be altered or the person counseled to deal with the environment effectively, the greater the probability of the treatment program producing sobriety.

The time has come for treatment programs to employ gerontologists with a sub-specialty of alcoholism training to provide for the needs of this unique population. The alcoholic over sixty must be identified and successfully treated in the large, multifaceted treatment program instead of being shuffled to other treatment (usually medical services). The elderly alcoholic is every bit a part of the problem-drinking population as the younger alcoholic. When the treatment outcome of these people demonstrates success, the referrals will increase and the prognosis will become much brighter.

One of the strongest stresses that can lead an elderly individual to begin drinking is the death of their spouse. Only rarely does an elderly married couple die at the same time. Often one is left to suffer the loneliness that has never been prepared for, anticipated, or thought about. The process of grieving for the death of a spouse in this age bracket is a minimum of two years. Many alcoholics in treatment in this age bracket have a case history that specifically pinpoints the death of the spouse as a time they lost control of their drinking. Statistically, men will be hit harder by the death of a wife than the wife is by the death of her husband. In this culture, it is understood that the woman will outlive the man by usually seven to ten years. Also, the man is more likely to die within two-and-one-half years of his mate's death than is a woman.

There is a void left in the lives of most retirees and widows that produces a combination of boredom, loneliness, uselessness, and despair. If these persist for longer than six months, then very often inadequacy, depression and a lack of self-esteem result. Each of these character defects are stepping stones to alcoholism. Treatment for this type of individual must be to reestablish and redefine life without the marital role. This is also much more often the man going through this process, since in this age bracket few housewives have ever had the opportunity to retire. Their work as housewives continues throughout their lifetime.

An important hazard to watch out for with the senior alcoholic is that of confusion in the taking of pills, whether prescribed or over the counter. A useful way of teaching recovery in alcoholics of this age to make sure they don't overdose on routine medication, during the initial parts of sobriety, is to buy one of the pillboxes that are available in most drugstores and lay out the day's medication according to the time that they will be taking it. Thus, they can check the pillbox and if the pills are there, they did not take them; if the pills are not there, they did take them. It is important to remember that an accidental overdose will kill an elderly person much more quickly and with fewer medications in that overdose than the younger counterpart.

The elderly alcoholic needs a physical a minimum of every six months to guarantee that the aftereffects of their drinking are not going untreated. A component of this exam is to determine that nutritional levels are adequate and that no disease process has gone unnoticed or undiagnosed. Also, the danger exists that diseases are overlooked in the early stage of recovery because a person requires time to recover and feel really good.

The issue of role reversal in getting the elderly alcoholic in treatment is also important to consider. The younger generation are told that they are to look up to, respect and not question their elders. Often, the elders have been called on to solve and settle problems and arguments among these younger persons. Because of this role, many younger persons, including the elderly alcoholic's own children, are unable to accept the fact that perhaps mom or dad has a drinking problem. This attitude encourages the elderly alcoholic to keep the habit hidden. If the children take any course at all, it is usually half-hearted and they normally make the same mistakes that they would make if any member of the family was an alcoholic. This role reversal usually causes a break in the family system and numerous resentments.

The elderly alcoholic does not want to be told by a child that alcohol has become a problem, that their drinking has gotten out of hand, and that they of all people might be injured by it. This is an especially difficult dilemma for the child who is a caretaker of the elderly drinker and who becomes an enabler for the drinker to continue drinking. When a family system such as this is encountered, it is important to treat the whole family system as would be the case with any younger alcoholic.

There are some important differences between the elderly alcoholic and their younger counterpart in the same treatment program. To deny that these exist is to make the program less effective in building sobriety for each of the age groups involved. With a shortage of community facilities and the lack of treatment know-how for problems specific to the elderly, some programs are not relevant to the needs of this population. Compounding this problem is the lack of personal resources or insurance benefits sufficient to secure the available services the aged person requires. Frequently, the problems and needs of these persons have been ignored by the service staffs of the programs in which these people become involved. The goal of sobriety in the sixty- plus age bracket is different and often misunderstood by treatment personnel. The goal in this age bracket is for the individual to become sober and to be able to manipulate their environment in the situations causing distress to them.

Transportation for treatment, as with other health care needs of the elderly, may be difficult or impossible. Another difference in the elderly alcoholic is the time required for successful detoxification. Insurance companies, including Medicare, have misunderstood that the older problem drinker will require more time to feel good and to withdraw from the addictive process before beginning treatment. Thus, where the younger counterpart may feel good in three or four days and be ready to begin a treatment program, it might be seven to ten days for the older alcoholic to feel well and be able to enter the treatment program. Thus, this means that the person only is able to utilize approximately half of whatever that treatment program consists of. Compounding this problem is that older, retired problem drinkers are often regarded as poor treatment risks. Agencies may feel, consciously or not, that resources are better spent on younger problem drinkers for whom rehabilitation may be identified by a return to employment.

Similiarities of treating the elderly and the other age groups are:

1. The concept of abstinence of alcohol being a key to recovery.
2. Rebuilding a life that is meaningful.
3. Rebuilding family relationships that still exist.
4. Problems of keeping and maintaining sobriety in a culture that values the right to drink.

The caring and concern that alcoholism treatment and Alcoholics Anonymous both provide can give the older alcoholic, who does not have a family, someone with which to be involved and thus make that person's life more rewarding. Self-help knows no age barrier, race barrier, or economic barrier. Often, the older alcoholic is able to make a significant impact on an alcoholic in the teens or early twenties and can, in fact, be instrumental in turning that person's life around for them. The whole issue of fellowship and concern can bring tremendous rewards for both individuals entering into that relationship.

Recovery means getting busy and staying involved with other people. The role of the senior citizen can be exciting and enjoyable if certain attitudes, such as negative thinking and pessimism towards other people, are changed. Volunteers in the alcohol unit that helped with sobriety, or volunteer work with the Alcoholics Anonymous group they want to attend, can be tremendously rewarding for the senior citizen. The senior citizen alumni groups of hospital-based programs have an ongoing and exciting role in those treatment programs. These people often become indispensable to the treatment staff because they have a large amount of time and enthusiasm to give. In communities with high senior citizen populations, an AA senior citizen group may even be appropriate.

Because individuals in the age category of sixty and up are conscious of the fact that little time probably exists in their life span, these alcoholics often recover much more quickly, achieve a much more satisfying sobriety, and maintain it with greater consistency than younger victims of alcoholism. Once this population is readily understood and treated with a consistency in all treatment programs, the rewards of treating this population will become self-evident. Because of the rapidly escalating number of persons in this age bracket, treating these people is no longer an option but is now a necessity.

Suicide

Twenty-five percent of all persons who commit suicide are over age sixty-five. The rate of suicide for persons over sixty-five is five times that of the general population. After age seventy-five, the rate is eight times higher. In working with the elderly, a suicide evaluation is not to be neglected, since so many depressions are masked in their appearance.

Practical Treatment Suggestions

Kenny and Leaton in their book, *Loosening The Grip,* provide some general guidelines for treatment personnel in dealing with the elderly.*

1. If the elderly have some symptoms of psychological problems or physical problems, including a problem with alcohol, provide the same treatment you would for someone younger. Too often,

---

*From Goodstein, Richard: Special populations: The Elderly. In Kinney, Jean, and Leaton, Gwen: *Loosening the Grip* (St. Louis, C.V. Mosby Co., 1978). Reproduced by permission.

problems of the elderly are dismissed under the assumption the elderly are just complainers, senile, unlikely to benefit, likely to die soon, or incapable of appreciating help.

2. In making an evaluation of an older person, do a comprehensive assessment rather than just a symptom-oriented search. Pay attention to the social, financial, emotional, medical, cognitive, and self-care status. The latter is often overlooked. Is the person able to do the daily activities required for well-being, such as preparing meals, getting groceries, taking medications, as prescribed?

3. Since many elderly persons are reluctant to seek or receive professional help, a family member is often the person to make the first contact. This will initially be your best source of information about the person. Be sure to find out the family's views of the situation, their ideas and fears. Whatever the problem, the chances are good that something can be done to improve the picture. Let the family know about this optimism. It often comes as a surprise to them that their elderly relative may get better.

4. Sometimes the family will appear to you as unhelpful, unsympathetic, or uncaring. This may infuriate and annoy you. Even if this happens, do not alienate the family. Whatever problems there may be with the family, it is possibly the only support system the client has.

5. In dealing with the elderly, remind yourself you are working with persons who are survivors. The fact that they have made it this far means they have some strengths. These people have stuck their necks out in the past and taken risks. Find out how they have done it and see if you can help them replicate that. Also, raise their expectations that indeed they can "make it" again, just as they have before.

6. Use all the possible resources at your disposal. In many instances the elderly need to become reinvolved in the world around them. Meaningful contacts can come from a variety of people, not just from professional helpers. The janitor in the client's apartment building, a neighbor, or a crossing guard at the street corner may all be potential allies. If the person was once active in a church group, civic organization, or other community group but has lost contact, get in touch with the organization. There is often a member who will visit or be able to assist in other ways. Many communities have senior citizen centers. They offer a wide range of resources; everything from a social program to Meals-on-Wheels, to counseling on Social Security and Medicare, to transportation. If there is a single agency to cultivate, this is the one.

7. In your interviews with the elderly, the importance of reaching out, showing interest, and having physical contact has already been mentioned. Also be active. Do not merely sit there and grunt from time to time. Your quietness may too easily be interpreted by them as distance and dislike. Another very important thing to do is to provide cues to orient the elderly. Mention dates, day of the week, current events. For anyone who has had any cognitive slippage, good cues from the environment are very helpful. In conversation with the elderly, don't stick with neutral topics like the weather all the time. Try to engage them in some topics of common interest to you both (such as gardening, baseball, etc.) as well as some controversial topic. Something with some zip stimulates their egos, since it implies that you not only want their opinions but you want them to listen to yours.

8. If you give specific information to the client, also write it down for him in legible handwriting. This makes it much easier for the client to comply. If family members are present, tell them the directions, too. In thinking about compliance and what can be done to assist the elderly in participating in treatment, take some time to think about how your agency functions. What does it mean for an elderly client coming to see you? Are there long waits at several different offices on several different floors? Does it require navigating difficult stairs, elevators, and hallways in the process? Are there certain times of the day that make the use of public transportation easier? Consider such factors and make adjustments to make it much easier for your elderly client. In specific terms, make every effort to do things in as uncomplicated, convenient, non-embarrassing and economical a fashion as possible.

9. Separate sympathy and empathy. Sympathy is feeling sorry for someone. The elderly do not want that as it makes them feel like children. Empathy means you understand or want to understand. This is what they would like.

10. Be aware that you may be thought of and responded to as any number of important people in your client's long life. Also, you may alternately represent grandchild, child, parent, peer, and authority figure to them at various points in treatment, even in the same interview and at the same time.

11. Display integrity with the elderly. Do not try to mislead them or lie to them. They are too experienced with all the con games in life. If they ask you questions, give them straight answers. This, however, does not mean being brutal in the name of honesty. For example, in speaking with a client you might well say, "Many other people I talk with have concerns about death, do you?" The client responds, "No, I have pretty much come to

terms with the idea of dying." You don't blurt out, "Well, you better think about it, you only have six months to live." That is not integrity.

12. In working with elderly clients, set specific goals. Make sure that the initial ones are easily attainable. This means they can have some surefire positive experiences. With that under their belts, they are more likely to take some risks and attempt other things.

13. Make home visits. Home visits are the key to working with this group. It may be the only thing that will break down their resistance and help them get treatment. Very few will seek help on their own initiative. So, if someone is not willing to come to your office, give them a call. Ask if you can make an appointment to see them at home. If the response you get is "I don't want you to come," don't quit. Your next line is, "Well, if I'm ever in the area, I'd like to stop by." And try to do that. Bring some small token gift, such as notepaper or flowers. After your visit, you may well find the resistance has disappeared.

The home visit can be vital in making an adequate assessment. Seeing the person in his own home, where security is at its peak, provides a much better picture of how the person is getting along, as well as the pluses and minuses of the environment. It also allows the patient to be spontaneous in emotions and behavior. If you regularly make home visits, beware of making the person "stay in trouble" in order to see you. Don't just visit in a crisis, but instead stop in to hear about successes. Your visits may be a real high point for the person, who may not like to think of losing this contact. Make a visit the day after the client's first day on a new volunteer job, for example.

14. Beware of arranging things for the elderly that will be seen as something trivial to occupy their time. If there is a crafts class, the point ought to be to teach them a skill, an art, not to keep them busy. Many of the elderly also have something they can teach others. The carpenter who is no longer steady enough to swing a hammer and drive a nail will be able to provide consultation to do-it-yourselfers who want to remodel their homes. The elderly have a richness of life experiences and much to contribute.

15. Thoroughly evaluate symptoms of memory loss, disorientation and behavioral changes to uncover potentially treatable causes of organic brain syndrome. Have patients show you all their medicines, including the over-the-counter types. Coordinate medical care to avoid duplication of prescriptions.

In closing, the task in working with the elderly is to assist them in rediscovering strengths, getting involved with people and discovering life is worth living at whatever age.

Chapter 9

TREATING ALCOHOLICS

Approaches to Treatment

ALL treatment programs and philosophies include certain components.

Individual Therapy. This approach allows individualized treatment goals and objectives and gives each person in the program individual therapy and attention.

Often this format is the most helpful for the elderly alcoholic since they may be unwilling to speak in a group. Many issues are raised and settled in this setting. Some treatment professionals are utilized frequently in this approach.

Group Therapy. By far the most common, groups are utilized extensively in all treatment programs. Groups are used for education, psychotherapy, films, lectures, discussions, guest speakers, AA, and numerous other purposes.

Often, in the group discussion, concerns are raised that affect several group members. Also, the group teaches folks to once again deal with other people's needs and concerns. Thus, resocialization occurs and friendships result.

Self-Help. That alcoholics (and their families) help new members to the group is a well-known fact. Often an alcoholic can allay another's fears or pain better than anyone else. Alcoholics Anonymous's phenomenal success bears this fact out.

Treatment staffs often learn a great deal by listening to their group members during coffee breaks and relaxed times. Usually when someone is not progressing, it is another alcoholic who is able to convince them that treatment works and is worthwhile.

Bibliotherapy. Alcoholics must understand that their recovery is their responsibility, not the treatment staff's, and thus hard work is required. One of the most advantageous approaches is bibliotherapy—an outside, therapeutic homework assignment. Those who receive and do their assignments are able to reach conclusions and learn apart from the therapist. Thus, they develop their own convictions, which strengthen them for stressful times. One reason this has not been used more often is that treatment staffs are not abreast of current literature. To assign a reading requires knowing what is contained in the reading.

The bibliotherapy guide at the end of this chapter does not purport to be complete. However, these booklets are informative, transcend most educational limitations, are cost effective, and are short enough to be of immediate assistance.

The alcoholic must develop an attitude of utilizing information in their recovery. Good reading material should be available to them at all times.

Family Groups. This subject is covered extensively in the next chapter. Suffice it to say that families need the same kinds of education as does the alcoholic. Thus, some coordination of information must occur.

Alcoholics Anonymous. Every treatment program exposes its clients to AA as part of their treatment program. Thus, misconceptions and questions can be handled during therapy. Some programs have run into AA groups who were negative towards a formal treatment program. Fortunately, such AA groups are in a minority. Many AA groups are treatment allies and provide immediate sponsors to those showing interest in AA. The AA program is discussed in greater detail in Chapter 11, "Self-Help Groups: Alcoholism Recovery."

Components of Therapy

Detoxification. Depending on the age of the alcoholic and the length and amount of drinking, detox requires anywhere from twenty-four hours to ten days. The average is three to five days.

The detoxification process is discussed in some detail in Chapter 5. "Medical and Physician's Issues." However, some key points to remember:

1. The alcoholic coming off a major episode will be sick and needs to be comforted by staff. The comfort received is the difference between whether the alcoholic stays or leaves against medical advice (AMA).
2. The more comfortable the patient is physically, the better the patient will do in the program.
3. Detox can be a major medical crisis requiring life-sustaining measures.

Education. Education is one of the major components of all treatment programs and centers on the disease of alcoholism and skills of daily living and problem solving.

How this is accomplished varies tremendously between programs but covers much the same information. This includes the disease concept, physiology, psychology of drinking behavior, nutrition, stress management and relapse indicators. Most programs utilize some combination of films, handouts, lectures and group discussions to accomplish this goal.

Personal Character Challenges. Each individual in treatment has some areas of their character that require examination and change. Most of these are involved in the person's addiction. These areas may involve honesty, assertiveness, decision-making skills, relationship skills and any number of emotional components.

The alcoholic must face the emotions which arise without chemical assistance. To do so means to begin identifying emotions and learning to cope with them.

Aftercare

Any successful aftercare program has to combine group therapy, some education, individual therapy and family therapy themes. Each setting is required to meet the multiplicity of issues the newly recovering must face.

Education. This might be more accurately called reemphasis of key educational components contained in the initial therapy. It is impossible for anyone to learn all that is offered in most treatment programs initially. Also once the alcoholic begins to apply the information supplied to his/her daily life-style, the information takes on new relevance. Thus, questions requiring clarification arise.

Individual Therapy. Some private sessions may be required, especially for persons who must reenter unstable homes or other stressful situations. Most agency/program staffing patterns prohibit this on a regular basis for every person, but the graduates of a program need to know that this is available to them.

Group Therapy. Most aftercare programs are run in a group format on either a weekly basis or a biweekly basis. Most issues facing the newly recovering alcoholic are dealt with in this setting. This has been, by far, the most effective.

Family Therapy. These groups are generally run concurrently with the alcoholic group. At times, circumstances may suggest combining the two groups to view a key movie or discuss a major development. The family group continually reinforces the need for all to recover.

Alumni Associations. For treatment programs, this approach has proven beneficial for both the programs and the individuals. It provides a ready pool of volunteers who can provide transportation, sit with a detox patient, go to a meeting with a new treatment client, or any of the other functions that were previously discussed. The alumni benefit tremendously by giving away their sobriety and gaining the continuing support of the staff. Alumni associations are being utilized by every major treatment program in some form.

Alcoholics Anonymous. Some persons have maintained that AA is the only ongoing aftercare program that works. The advantage of AA is that meetings are usually available wherever the alcoholic is. However, AA is not the only aftercare program, especially for the elderly. Whatever has worked for the person is what should be followed.

Treatment Impairment Wheel

This unique tool is a self-report treatment planning instrument. Tests have indicated that it is most useful in allowing alcoholics of all backgrounds, ages and educational levels to have opportunity to report on how they perceive their problems.

The impairment wheel is presented in Figure 9-1. The wheel asks each person to assess the twelve major areas of functioning. The rating scale is based on simple percentages (e.g. 25%, 50%,

75%, 100%). The question is, How much of the time has alcohol caused impairment in the area of _____ .

IMPAIRMENT WHEEL.

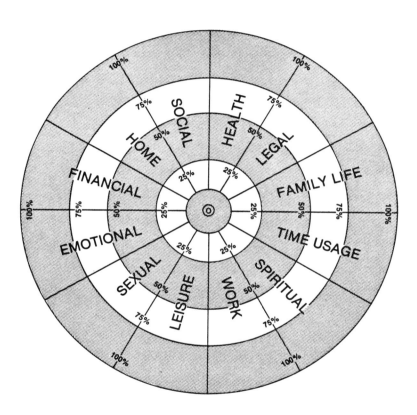

AGE   SEX   RACE   MARITAL STATUS   LENGTH OF SOBRIETY

Figure 9-1. The impairment wheel is a simple tool that facilitates client feedback in the treatment process. The client evaluates each major life area according to the percentage of time alcohol use intervenes.

The self-report should be completed early in the treatment process and can be used to isolate degree of denial, issues that are of concern and gives the individual the opportunity to express their opinion of treatment issues.

By using such an item in treatment planning, the client often devotes self to treatment because of a say in treatment. Research has indicated this is vital to successful treatment.

Older alcoholics (over age 50) tested above 50 percent consistently in the areas of financial, spiritual, health and leisure. Younger alcoholics tended to isolate work, time, family and sexual issues.

The advantage of the treatment impairment wheel over the checklist method is the absence of troublesome phrases and the major area report.

Other Treatment Issues

A bias that treatment individuals need to carefully guard against is that of giving more attention or more therapy time to the younger alcoholic than to the elderly alcoholic. This is not an unnatural bias. Even in the medical field, often a doctor will sustain life much more ambitiously in a young patient than he will an elderly patient. The quality of life for a senior citizen is certainly no less satisfying or rewarding than it is for a younger person in treatment. Often an unwritten factor is that of the person being in later years and, thus, the productivity expectation is less for that individual as opposed to a younger person who has career, wife, and children for a good many years ahead of him. Again, this is an area that is not considered carefully enough, and in a treatment setting the elderly alcoholic is keenly aware that hereto they are second-class citizens and not as vital as the young around them. Although the treatment approaches for the young vary from the treatment approaches for the elderly, they are no less rewarding and no less obligatory for the treating professionals or the treating agency. The stigma attached to being old must be overcome in the professional's attitude before there is any hope of helping the client overcome it in their life.

Still another controversy currently being debated is within the field of alcoholism treatment. The debate centers on medical detox as opposed to social-setting detoxes. When considering this argument, the first point is the old adage that if the alcoholic suffers enough during withdrawal, he will not return to drinking. This is a throwback to the punitive approach to the alcoholic that he should suffer for the addiction that he has undergone.

Professionals and families alike tend to approach the alcoholic requesting confirmation, "I am an alcoholic," as though the simple admission to the fact will cure the disease. It is unrealistic expectations like these that must be overcome if there is to be any hope for the person to not only achieve sobriety but maintain it for any significant length of time.

Obviously, the admission "I am an alcoholic" or "I have a disease" is but the very minutest portion of the building block on which sobriety is built. Some research in the field has indicated that people who come in and say that "drinking has caused me a problem" and classify themselves as a problem drinker but never do say "I am an alcoholic" are apt to recover and do just as well as those who do, but the admission needs to be alcohol has caused me a problem, not "I am an alcoholic" per se.

The whole issue of denial has always been an interesting one. At the core of any abusive kind of behavior is the lack of self-love. People who hammer and hammer at an alcoholic, or the alcoholic addicted, wanting that admission and wanting them to admit that they are powerless and they've lost control need to be standing there to pick up those pieces when the roof caves in, as it will. That admission will always bring about the mourning of a lost friend, even though that lost friend is alcohol.

For the elderly, that loss is even more significant than perhaps it is for a younger person who still has family, job and a good social-support system. In older age when often family has either died or moved, retirement has come, and loss of status in terms of financial functioning and independence have come, there may be some ill health, and losing alcohol may become another profound loss and one that people often choose not to give up.

Values

A major point in treatment strategy is before we decide what is best for the client, we best check with the client first. For example, to tell people that sexual behavior, including masturbation, homosexuality, and sleeping with persons other than your spouse, is all right when in fact it conflicts with the person's interbeing and values is to set them up for still another conflict for which they might be ill equipped to deal with. We, instead, in treatment must encourage people to act according to their values. Should those values be contradictory or not functional in the client's life at the time, then values clarification may very well be in order. However, a client should never be told that it is all right to act contradictory to their values, since this sets them up for failure and more problems.

Denial

Most professionals treat the statement by an elderly alcoholic that "Drinking is all I have to live for" as a form of denial. This is perhaps the most serious mistake that the professional can make in the treatment of an elderly alcoholic. The alcoholic who has lost job, spouse, children, perhaps has health problems and has had to accept a lower standard of living truly may not have a great deal to live for. It is imperative that this be seen as a warning sign of impending hopelessness and desire to die as opposed to denial.

If seen that way, then the treatment plan is obvious. It becomes one of helping the person to reestablish healthy life patterns that perhaps they either don't know how to do or don't have the ego strength to do. This involves rebuilding the person's motivation and helping him to establish a disciplined pattern of living that includes nutrition, sleep, recreation and social activities. In the urban setting, this might be as simple as involving him/her in a senior citizen center activity in the neighborhood. A word of caution on that approach is that the person will rarely follow through on attending the senior citizen center alone, which is not surprising since most of us don't go to a place where we know none of the people. Thus, it is imperative to have a volunteer or someone who can help that person make friends and feel adjusted in that setting.

The case of Mr. T is a good example.

As a seventy-four-year-old alcoholic in treatment, he literally has no family except for one duaghter who lived in the north, no friends, was living in a semi-tenement-type housing development, literally lived paycheck to paycheck on Social Security, and had little or no contact with the outside world. Upon discharge from treatment, he was referred to his neighborhood senior citizen center.

Unfortunately, because he did not know anybody and was hesitant to reach out and trust people he did not know, he never followed through on that referral. Predictably, within two weeks he was drinking. The drinking binge lasted for approximately three weeks when he again had to be entered into detox in a medically unstable condition.

The case of Mr. T is neither surprising nor unusual. Again, it is imperative that these people be introduced into new social settings with someone they can trust that has visited them and who knows them and who can introduce them around and help them not to feel unwanted or out of place. This is one of the most excellent uses of a volunteer program: to have folks who will visit these alcoholics in their home who will bond to them as friends and who will introduce them into a senior citizen center, church activities or perhaps even sporting events, depending on the person's interest.

In the rural setting, it is much more difficult to rebuild a social base of support for the elderly alcoholic. In the rural setting, transportation is often a major obstacle in even getting the person into treatment in the first place. Ongoing treatment is often impossible unless there is a volunteer who can intervene and provide that transportation for the individual. In most rural areas even though the population of elderly may be high, transportation and logistics often prohibit the development of senior citizen centers. Thus, the choices for rebuilding social support are often limited to the immediate community around that individual. This usually means a church group, a recreation center, a congregate meal site or some other such program.

Many agencies have found it necessary to have a gerontology outreach program, where volunteers are trained to go into the homes of these individuals and provide friendship and companionship, as well as transportation to medical appointments and other such needs for the elderly person. This is an excellent program approach for those years in which funding is difficult and resources are limited.

Probably this affects, in a rural setting, a woman alcoholic or the spouse of an alcoholic much more severely than it does a male in the same setting. Rural women tend to be much less mobile than do their counterparts in the urban setting. Men will generally be able to get where they want to go, but women generally do not find that resource available.

Relapse Guide

Any treatment for a major medical problem indicates some instruction of how to know if recovery is not on schedule. Surgery patients are instructed on care of sutures, cleansing the wound, elevation and so forth; chemotherapy patients are instructed as to side effects and dosage requirements; and alcoholics must be instructed on relapse. No alcoholic just begins drinking for no reason. Measurable and answerable behaviors and attitudes always precede the first drink.

Probably, the most valid criticism of treatment programs is the lack of emphasis on relapse. If the bulk of the teaching about relapse is left for the aftercare component of the program, this will be too late for some. Since no cure exists for alcoholism, the individual must begin each day by preparing against the dangers that will arise daily.

The major components of the dry drunk syndrome and the relapse potential are presented in Figures 9-2 and 9-3. The difference between dry drunk and relapse is marginal in most professionals' opinions. However, there is one major differentiation: the dry drunk attitudes and behaviors may go on for some period of time (months or years in rare cases) before the first drink is taken. The dry drunk is defined as a return to the attitudes and behaviors that characterized the individual's life while drinking. The return is most always in subtle ways, which are almost imperceptable at first. By the time the individual is obviously in trouble, many of his/her attitudes are prohibitive of intervention.

The Progression and Recovery of the Alcoholic in the Disease of Alcoholism

To be read from left to right.

Progression

Occasional Relief Drinking
Constant Relief Drinking Commences

Crucial Phase

Urgency of First Drinks
Feelings of Guilt
Memory Blackouts Increase
Drinking Bolstered with Excuses
Grandiose and Aggressive Behavior
Efforts to Control Fail Repeatedly
Tries Geographical Escapes
Family and Friends Avoided
Loss of Ordinary Will Power

Increase in Alcohol Tolerance
Onset of Memory Blackouts
Surreptitious Drinking
Increasing Dependence on Alcohol
Unable to Discuss Problem
Decrease of Ability to Stop Drinking When Others Do So
Persistent Remorse
Promises and Resolutions Fail
Loss of Other Interests
Work and Money Troubles
Unreasonable Resentments
Neglect of Food
Physical Deterioration

Chronic Phase

Tremors and Early Morning Drinks
Decrease in Alcohol Tolerance
Onset of Lengthy Intoxications
Moral Deterioration
Impaired Thinking
Drinking with Inferiors
Indefinable Fears
Unable to Initiate Action
Obsession with Drinking
Vague Spiritual Desires
All Alibis Exhausted
Complete Defeat Admitted

Obsessive Drinking Continues in Vicious Circles

Rehabilitation

Honest Desire for Help
Learns Alcoholism is an Illness
Told Addiction Can Be Arrested
Stops Taking Alcohol
Meets Normal and Happy Former Addicts
Takes Stock of Self
Right Thinking Begins
Spiritual Needs Examined
Physical Overhaul by Doctor
Onset of New Hope
Start of Group Therapy
Appreciation of Possibilities of New Way of Life
Diminishing Fears of the Unknown Future
Return of Self-Esteem
Desire to Escape Goes
Adjustment to Family Needs
New Interests Develop
Rebirth of Ideals
Appreciation of Real Values
Confidence of Employers
Contentment in Sobriety
Increasing Tolerance

Regular Nourishment Taken
Realistic Thinking
Natural Rest and Sleep
Family and Friends Appreciate Efforts
New Circle of Stable Friends
Facts Faced with Courage
Increase of Emotional Control
Economic Stability
Care of Personal Appearance
First Steps Towards
Rationalizations Recognized

Recovery

Group Therapy and Mutual Help Continue

Enlightened and Interesting Way of Life Opens Up with Road Ahead to Higher Levels than Ever Before

Courtesy of
CareUnit® Program
Comprehensive Care Corporation

© 1982 **CompCare** publications

Figure 9-2. A tool to diagnose all of the various components of the disease as well as the components of recovery. (Copyright© 1982, CompCare Publications, 2415 Annapolis Lane, Minneapolis, Minnesota 55441. Reproduced by permission.)

RELAPSE POTENTIAL©		
RELAPSE IMMINENT	**RELAPSE PROBABLE**	**RELAPSE POSSIBLE**
Other Mood Altering Chemicals Surreptitious Light Drinking Know-It-All Attitude Contentious Attitude Cockiness Blaming Others Withdrawal from Others Emotionally Grandiosity Isolation	Careless Choice of Places Ingratitude Complacency Frustration Exhaustion Boredom With Recovery Program Careless Use of Time Self-Pity Dishonesty	Unrealistic Goals Physical Illness Poor Priorities Impatience Euphoria Depression Unexplained Anxiety Worry, Pride Too Serious Fear

Figure 9-3. This tool gives an overview of the potential for relapse when these characteristics are left unchanged or allowed to recur.

Characteristics of Imminent Relapse

1. *Surreptitious, light drinking*: This is also known as maintenance drinking and sneak drinking. How long any individual can drink lightly before escalating back into binge drinking varies greatly. However, unless intervention occurs, the individual will be back to square one in the recovery program. The light drinker is usually different from the person who gives in during a situation for which preparation was not made in advance. The light drinker is knowingly trying "to beat the odds." This says much about the overall changes required.

2. *Use of Mood-Altering Chemicals*: This is often insidious for the elderly, because often the mood-altering chemical is a prescription medication given by a physician. The most dangerous drugs prescribed are Valium, Librium, Dalmane, and certain of the medications used to alleviate anxiety and depression. Of course, in younger alcoholics and in certain elderly alcoholics, marijuana and many of the street drugs are used. Treatment must include education on uses of all these drugs and their implication for relapse. The more stress placed on this danger and the

non-chemical alternatives, the better the chance for not falling into the danger.

3. *Know-It-All Attitude*: This always guarantees major difficulties. The person who cannot be instructed and sees no need to listen or learn from others will not survive. Treatment teams end up in combative sessions when these persons come to treatment. Often, this is a major problem in DWI schools and for individuals who are court-ordered in for treatment. A combination of caring and confrontation by treatment staffs can help the person overcome this attitude, especially if the person is reacting this way out of fear and insecurity. "I already know that" is often a reason given for not wanting to continue AA and aftercare. Being reminded helps each person remember how bad drinking can be.

4. *Contentious Attitude*: Treating the "pseudo-prosecuter" is always enjoyable. This person openly scoffs at information and refuses to take any teaching at face value. If the treatment staff remains patient and convinces the person, then the client usually will do well.

In aftercare and AA, this attitude must be confronted each time it appears. Treatment staff may first become aware that this is a problem when informed by family members of related difficulties at home.

5. *Cockiness*: This is one of the most observable. The individual's demeanor becomes one of exaggerated confidence (à la the strut). The person will refer to themself as "recovered," instead of "recoving," and will brag about all the bars they frequent without being affected by the drinking. This individual may even go so far as to be host of a well-stocked bar and brag as to being a top-notch bartender. The fall will be hard.

6. *Blaming Others*: Each person alive makes mistakes daily. Some are more serious than others. To embark on a course of denying mistakes and blaming others is a major danger sign.

This may show itself in subtle ways such as finger pointing at people who try to point out mistakes. Again, the family can be most helpful in alerting the staff that this is happening.

7. *Withdrawal from Others Emotionally*: Alcoholism is a disease with a major emotional component. One of the major complaints of the spouse is that the alcoholic is unable to give of themselves emotionally.

When the alcoholic begins recovery, often the feelings are new to them. This is particularly true of the alcoholic with a long course of drinking. Opening oneself up is difficult, painful and costly. Much time must be devoted in encouraging discussion of hurts that will invariably arise, especially in a marriage.

Also, be aware of what the individual considers normal. Many strive to be normal but have a highly unrealistic idea of what normal is.

8. *Grandiosity*: No one person is going to save the world, convert mankind to a given cause, or sober up all alcoholics. Yet, some individuals act as if they can do all of this. This type of behavior is usually to cover up a lack of self-respect and character defects. Such people are difficult to help until they open themselves up some.

9. *Isolation*: This is the major cause of relapse for the elderly. Too much time alone guarantees allowing weaknesses to rise to the surface. Such unhealthy tendencies cannot be given time to fester.

Characteristics of Probable Relapse

1. *Careless Choice of Places*: Non-drinkers have very little business being in a lounge or bar at any time for any reason. To go into such places is to wear down defenses and to allow the drink to become desirable. The possible exception to this is the AA member doing twelve-step work, or the treatment staff recovering alcoholic attempting to assist a program member.

2. *Ingratitude*: Loss of motivation to work at recovery, marriage, child rearing and career can be traced to not being grateful for the blessings of having all those things and people. For example, a widow/widower will become immediately impatient with someone expressing resentments towards their spouse.

Consideration and meditation on what someone has changed from will result in two things: first, not slipping back into those qualities that were destructive; secondly, seeing changes encourages them to go forward and continue to change.

3. *Complacency*: Alcoholism does not lend itself to a "let up and coast" kind of approach. Day-to-day work is required for sobriety to have lasting value.

4. *Frustration*: This can range from minor irritations (such as a car pulling out in front of the person) to major frustrations. All can have a cumulative effect and result in short tempers and a "what's the use in trying" attitude.

5. *Exhaustion*: Although all careers at times result in effort beyond the normal workweek, exhaustion cannot and must not be the rule. If tired all the time (and nothing is physically wrong), then the individual must reassess their priorities. Learning to say no to less important demands is vital. The elderly must realize the need to pace themselves. No one functions well when they are too tired to think.

6. *Boredom with Recovery Program*: Boredom generally results from a combination of pride and not setting goals. The goals need to enter into all phases of the person's life. For example:

Financial: Pay off hospital bill.

AA: Contact sponsor daily at 6:00 PM

Church: Attend on a regular basis.

Family: Attend the reunion in three weeks.

Grandchildren: Take to zoo as promised.

Goals need not bog a person down hopelessly. However, the goals need to be set and acted upon. Self-worth is increased and satisfaction results from accomplishing the little things *every day.*

7. *Careless Use of Time*: Wasting time without plans is highly detrimental to any person at any time. Relaxation is vital, but not to extremes. Scheduling can and should be part of people's regular life. If the individual has large blocks of time left unaccounted for, then some planning and activity must be found (a major problem for the elderly). Busy for busy's sake is frustration. However, many are just stuck and don't know how to be involved.

8. *Self-Pity*: This is the "poor me" and "no one has it as hard as me" attitude and is the predecessor of resentment and bitterness of those who seem to be doing better. Neither the alcoholic nor the elderly are alone in their plight. Self-pity is destructive.

9. *Dishonesty*: The little white lies are as devastating to the recovering alcoholic as any behavior can be. However, the honesty may need to be first with an AA sponsor or counselor if the family has not engaged in treatment. This fact is increasingly obvious

when applied to the individual's behavior while drinking. Many revelations must be carefully considered as to whether the family will be further injured by knowing.

Characteristics of Possible Relapse

1. *Unrealistic Goals*: Sobriety that is attempted without goals is due to failure. Likewise, goals must be measurable, specific and realistic. Goals should be built, in part, according to priorities that are set in treatment. Goals must include the building blocks by which the goal will be achieved. For example, if the goal for a man is to improve his marriage, then the building blocks might include a weekend pass to enable him to take her to dinner. He may need to buy her flowers, take her to a favorite restaurant, help her buy a new dress, or any of the niceties that are otherwise lost in drinking. The time frame should be fairly specific.

2. *Physical Illness*: Any major illness or chronic pain can render a person defenseless against most of the other stresses that an elderly person faces. Many alcoholics who do well against all other problems and stresses fail to deal with failing health. Major illnesses such as heart attack, stroke and cancer are completely devastating and often lead to drinking.

If any of the difficulties are a result of the alcoholism, the guilt and anguish are often unbearable.

3. *Poor Priorities*: Time that is poorly spent is one of the major contributors to unintentional relapse. The process involved is basic. Whenever someone fails to plan time and finances, their mind seems to wander into whatever the personal difficulty is, whether food, alcohol, cigarettes, etc. Once the mind arrives, the actions are sure to follow. Even times of relaxation can be structured to be enjoyable and yet be structured to prohibit this kind of relapse.

4. *Impatience*: The old cliché "Rome was not built in a day" applies to all addicted persons. Despite years of abuse and carelessness, the alcoholic wants a cure today, the dieter wants to lose ten pounds today, and the smoker wants to quit today.

Just as becoming an alcoholic is a process, so too is sobriety a process. Building a lasting sobriety is time-consuming and difficult. There are times of wanting more than a person can have. The test is, are you making steady progress?

5. *Euphoria*: Literature documents this as an obstacle to be watched. This must be differentiated from the happiness and satisfaction that come from recovery and reordering one's life. Euphoria can present itself as a manic stage or as a giddy kind of high. Some mood swings do occur with sobriety and are normal.

6. *Depression*: As with euphoria, bouts with depression are fairly common and no cause for major concern. As with all emotions, depression can have many causes and needs to be recognized as normal in many cases. Generally, most depression occurs because of a major stress or unpleasant event and disappears within a few hours to a few days. Any lingering depression needs to be discussed with the treatment staff.

7. *Unexplained Anxiety and Worry*: This is often expressed in terms of a fatalistic expectation. When life improves at home and at work, many often expect some catastrophe to occur. If, after gentle probing, no apparent cause is found, then gentle reassurance should be given.

8. *Pride*: A difference exists between confidence and cockiness, and between aggressiveness and assertiveness. As with all major life changes, an excitement will occur. This must not turn into an "I've got it made" attitude.

9. *Too Serious*: This is a major obstacle to the enjoyment of life. While achieving sobriety needs to be taken seriously, it must not become burdensome. Humor is a vital ingredient to successful living. To laugh at oneself and circumstances around them is to produce a healthier emotional life.

This practitioner has always enjoyed the patients' forming friendships and then playing pranks on each other and the staff. People must learn to enjoy themselves and each other. At times, when depression seemed to have set in for several group members, this therapist would ask them to share a funny event that maybe one of their children (or grandchildren) had done. Depression disappears quickly with a good belly laugh. Some of the group assignments were to read the comics and find one which referred to themselves or their families. The choices were wonderful! Having fun and enjoying oneself and those around you is vital to good health.

10. *Fear*: People are afraid of many things. The issue is whether the fears are realistic and whether someone is controlled by fear. Most elements of fear can be dealt with through obtaining information and solving issues.

Each of these twenty-eight areas have caused relapses in patients at times. Some bounced back quickly and some have not. Relapses are not the end of the world. Some assessment of when and how the person relapsed is essential. Most relapses are due to a bad choice or putting oneself in a bad situation. Thus, they are experiential and can be learned from with other's help.

The individual's disappointment about drinking must not be allowed to overwhelm the person. Most people who relapse are sober one year from the date of treatment. All major programs document that anywhere from 60 percent to 90 percent of their treatment graduates are sober after one year (although some percentage will have a short relapse).

Openness about drinking is the key to circumventing a binge or a return to the old pattern of drinking.

BIBLIOTHERAPY FOR ALCOHOLICS

Carle, Cecil E.: *Letters to Elderly Alcoholics.* Center City, Minnesota: Hazelden, 1980.

Gust, Dodie: *Up, Down, and Sideways on Wet and Dry Booze.* Minneapolis: CompCare, 1977.

Hegarty, Carol: *Alcoholism Today: The Progress and the Promise.* Minneapolis: CompCare, 1979.

Wegscheider, Don: *If Only My Family Understood Me.* Minneapolis: CompCare, 1979.

Wegscheider, Sharon: *The Family Trap.* Minnesota: Nurturing Networks, 1976.

SUGGESTED READINGS FOR
PROFESSIONALS WORKING WITH THE ALCOHOLIC

Alcoholics Anonymous: *The Big Book,* 3rd Ed. New York: Alcoholics Anonymous World Services, Inc., 1976

Kinney, Jean, and Leaton, Gwen: *Loosening the Grip: A Handbook of Alcohol Information.* St. Louis: C.V. Mosby Company, 1978.

Chapter 10

FAMILY TREATMENT

Development of Family Therapy

A LCOHOLISM affects the families of the victim as severely as the victim. Clinical treatment of alcoholism must deal with the family if the person is to recover. The literature in the field has long held that a child of an alcoholic has twice the risk than the child of a non-alcoholic to develop the disease. Added to this phenomenon are the spouses of alcoholics who manifest many of the same symptoms as the individual drinking. This was a major reason for the argument of the psychological manifestations of the disease. Some have argued that the spouse has the psychological makeup to become an alcoholic, but *was not* drinking.

Then a significant treatment breakthrough was made by Sharon Wegscheider, then of the Johnson Institute and now president of On-Site Training and Consulting, Inc. Mrs. Wegscheider determined that clinical manifestations of the illness in the family followed set roles most of the time, and her magnificent work has identified the roles the alcoholic and the family members adopt as the disease progresses (see Figure 10–1). Clinical practice validates this model and facilitates the treatment of the real needs of each of the members of the family. Mrs. Wegscheider's work should be mandatory reading for each professional in Alcoholism and Mental Health settings.

Alcoholism and the Family / Putting the Pieces Together

ROLE	BEHAVIORS	SELF WORTH	NEEDS
CHEMICALLY DEPENDENT PERSON	perfectionistic grandiose aggressive righteous, no mistakes charming blaming	shame inadequacy guilt	confrontation support accountability loved accepted
THE CHIEF ENABLER	super-responsible martyr — others first fragile sickly powerless compliant manipulative	anger guilt tired	support self-care confrontation expression of feeling
THE FAMILY HERO	successful performs well independent seeks approval perceptive helpful	guilt inadequacy	allow mistakes take risks vulnerability express feelings
THE SCAPEGOAT	sullen defiant acting out chemical use blaming	hurt at not being heard loneliness	support of feelings confrontation acceptance challenge to be listened to
THE LOST CHILD	creative loners solitary withdrawn	loneliness rage	invitation consistency encouragement rewards for efforts
THE MASCOT	hyperactive humor clumsy center of attention	fear of not belonging fear of breaking down	physical touch taken seriously information asked for input

Figure 10-1. This figure will help identify the various roles and behaviors that the alcoholic assumes, an evaluation of the alcoholic's self-worth in accordance with these, and the needs that the alcoholic must have for "putting the pieces together." (From an article by Sharon Wegscheider that appeared in *Alcoholism: The National Magazine*, 1(3):38, 1981. Courtesy of *Alcoholism* magazine.)

The other major breakthrough in family treatment was the development of the progression of the disease by CompCare (see Figure 10-2). This tool can be used in several ways. One is to utilize this as a diagnostic tool to convince the family of their need

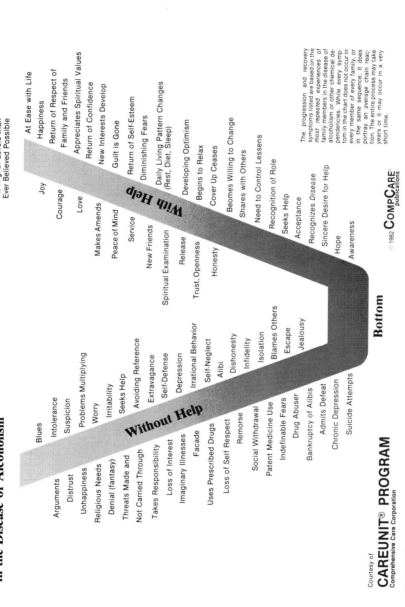

The Progression and Recovery of the Family in the Disease of Alcoholism

Courtesy of
CAREUNIT® PROGRAM
Comprehensive Care Corporation

Without Help

With Help

Bottom

Enlightened, Future Bright, to Higher Levels than Ever Believed Possible

At Ease with Life
Happiness
Return of Respect of Family and Friends
Appreciates Spiritual Values
Return of Confidence
New Interests Develop
Guilt is Gone
Return of Self-Esteem
Diminishing Fears
Daily Living Pattern Changes (Rest, Diet, Sleep)
Developing Optimism
Begins to Relax
Cover Up Ceases
Becomes Willing to Change
Shares with Others
Need to Control Lessens
Recognition of Role
Seeks Help
Acceptance
Recognizes *Disease*
Sincere Desire for Help
Hope
Awareness

Joy
Courage
Love
Makes Amends
Service
Peace of Mind
New Friends
Spiritual Examination
Release
Trust, Openness
Honesty

Blues
Intolerance
Suspicion
Problems Multiplying
Worry
Irritability
Seeks Help
Avoiding Reference
Extravagance
Self-Defense
Depression
Irrational Behavior
Self-Neglect
Alibi
Dishonesty
Infidelity
Isolation
Blames Others
Escape
Jealousy

Arguments
Distrust
Unhappiness
Religious Needs
Denial (fantasy)
Threats Made and
Not Carried Through
Takes Responsibility
Loss of Interest
Imaginary Illnesses
Facade
Uses Prescribed Drugs
Remorse
Loss of Self Respect
Social Withdrawal
Patent Medicine Use
Indefinable Fears
Drug Abuser
Bankruptcy of Alibis
Admits Defeat
Chronic Depression
Suicide Attempts

The progression and recovery symptoms listed are based on the *most repeated experiences* of family members in the disease of alcoholism or other chemical dependencies. While every symptom in the chart does not occur in every member of every family, or in the same sequence, it does portray an *average* chain reaction. The entire process may take years or it may occur in a very short time.

©1982 **CompCare** publications

Figure 10–2. This tool may be used for diagnosing symptoms of the family disease process and recovery. (Copyright© 1982, CompCare Publications, 2415 Annapolis Lane, Minneapolis, Minnesota 55441. Reproduced by permission.)

for treatment. When this is utilized in this manner, the educational value of the chart becomes obvious. Secondly, the chart can be used to teach the alcoholic how the family has been affected during the course of his/her alcoholism. Thus, meaningful dialogue between family members is facilitated.

The other overall value of both tools is to teach professionals in all fields of human services the progressive nature of family dysfunction. Once this has been understood, the problems of treatment modality and diagnosis are solved.

Enablers

Enablers are those persons who say and act in ways that allow the chemical abuser to continue chemical abuse. Most of the time, it is a person close to the abuser and who may have the best of intentions.

No alcoholic or anyone else will change as long as they escape the consequences of their addiction. People who chronically rescue the person and fix their crisis will enable the person to get worse. Because the enablers always are numbered among family members, combatting this process is difficult. Yet, much of the family illness stems from the stress of living binge to binge and crisis to crisis.

Enablers must change several areas to break out of the enabler role:

1. Understand that the alcoholic's consequences are his/hers alone to face. The alcoholic is the only one responsible (assuming the alcoholic is of legal age).
2. Allow the person to face the full consequences of their drinking behavior.
3. The non-enabler has the attitude that has been referred to as "tough love." The love is not rescuing someone from a little crisis so as to allow them to die of alcoholism.
4. When a crisis does occur, stop, think and act, instead of react.
5. Make no excuses on behalf of the alcoholic. Let the alcoholic make their own.
6. Do seek help to understand the process of addiction and to facilitate recovery for the whole family.

Myths Families Believe

Some myths of family treatment, particularly of the spouse, must be examined:

1. *"If I Stay, the Alcoholic will Quit Drinking."* This is probably not so. Often, the longer the family tolerates the drinking, the sicker the whole family becomes.

When the spouse threatens the drinker and does not follow through, then the more arrogant the drinker becomes. Even in a near stupor, the alcoholic knows, "I'm in control." When the spouse is the woman, she only becomes more terrified, isolated and sick. Especially for the elderly, mobility belongs to the man.

The wife may fully believe that to leave is to violate every value and belief she cherishes; thus, she stays and suffers.

2. *"If I do Leave, I'll Lose Everything."* Rarely is this the truth. Often, the male alcoholic threatens and bullies his wife into staying with this statement. Professionals must deal with this logically and gently. Few courts will ever find in favor of a male alcoholic who refuses to help himself. This is especially true if he is abusive. The wife will require extensive counseling before she leaves, if ever. For the wife who is unable or unwilling to leave, then helping her build a life-style in addition to her marriage will be the key to her mental health.

Even though the divorce rate in the United States is soaring, this has included few of the marriages in the over-sixty age bracket. These spouses truly made a lifetime commitment to their marriage partner. To even suggest to such a person that leaving the marriage is an option is seen as ridiculous and unrealistic. Thus, support, education and rebuilding the social structure are the components of therapy with these spouses.

3. *"Doesn't My Asking for Help Mean the Problem is Mine?"* Yes, to some extent. But the healthiest person in the family needs to initiate therapy for themselves and the other family members. Alcoholism in a family member means everyone will be affected who is close to the alcoholic.

Few people ever give much thought to alcoholism until personally confronted with the disease. To become involved with Al-Anon or a trained professional often means stopping the progression before the family is permanently altered by the pattern.

4. *"The Alcoholic Must Hit Bottom Before Being Helped."* Early in the history of alcoholism treatment, this was true. Now, this is not true. The Johnson Institute pioneered intervention as a method of raising the bottom up to the alcoholic. Virtually all treatment programs are now training personnel in this technique.

The process of Intervention is as follows:

A. Alcohol addiction and/or addiction to other drugs (often prescription drugs for the elderly) is determined to be the problem. Often, the family becomes so confused that they may be unsure on what to blame the problem. The addicted person's world becomes surrealistic, and the family must break out of this kind of world. Professionals can help to determine if the problem is alcoholism.

B. Once alcoholism is isolated as the problem, then the family must begin by working with themselves. *The family cannot do an intervention unless they work through their own feelings first.*

By beginning their own recovery first, they remove the biggest obstacle to successful intervention. Through settling their own feelings, the frustration turns to honesty and support towards the alcoholic. The intervention will produce resentment and anger in the alcoholic (usually only during the initial moments) and the family must be well enough to not respond to these emotions.

Also, in this phase of preparation, those who will provide the intervention must be identified. These are often family members but also may include clergymen, physician, attorney and employer.

When the person is elderly, the children may not live locally. However, most can obtain their training through a local center before going to the intervention.

C. The third step is to gather the specific information to be presented in the intervention setting. Each person who will participate in the intervention is asked to prepare a list of the dates, times, specific drinking behaviors encountered and the feelings and consequences of those behaviors on the person.

Samples from lists for each of the persons who might be present are given so that those who have not witnessed an intervention might familiarize themselves with how to structure statements. The alcoholic receiving the intervention is John:

Spouse: Honey, I love you. On the third of May, you came into my 2:00 PM bridge group very intoxicated. You called me a stupid whore with nothing better to do when I asked why you were home early. I was so upset, I cried an hour.

Child: Dad, you know I love you and respect you. On the second of March, I asked for the car keys so I could go to the store for mom. You had been drinking, so you slapped me. I was hurt and disappointed.

Attorney: John, you came to me as your attorney and friend in April because of being arrested for DWI. Because I care, I plea-bargained a lighter sentence for you. John, you had been drinking prior to the hearing. I'm upset and concerned for you.

Minister: John, two Sundays ago, you came to services for the first time in almost a year. We were so pleased, although you were obviously battling a hangover. But John, you sang almost a full verse after the song ended. I was embarrassed for you and your family. I'm here to help you because I care for you.

Physician: John, I have been your doctor for five years. You came in for a checkup last month and I ran some tests. Your BAL was 0.15 at 3:00 PM, yet you did not appear drunk. Your liver profile indicates cirrhosis of the liver has begun; yet, you deny these are signs of addiction. You will die within a year without treatment.

Employer: John, you've worked here for over ten years. On the third of June, you came back from lunch one-and-one-half hours late and were so intoxicated I drove you home. I care about you, but you must get treatment in order to keep your job. I'll be here to help all I can.

Neighbor: John, I've been your friend for ten years. You helped me tremendously when my wife was so sick last year. On the second of July, you ran over my mailbox and hit the garbage cans at 3:00 AM. John, your drinking has taken you over.

The essence of intervention: the drinker's behavior is presented factually with ample love, support and concern. Although the drinker may begin with anger and defensiveness, this is broken by the love and concern of those who love him/her. Oftentimes, the person will be so overwhelmed that time will need to be provided for crying and hugging as well as thinking.

The second phase of the intervention is the goal: get the alcoholic into a formal treatment program. Part of the preparation for the intervention is to explore available treatment and to make all entry arrangements prior to the time of the intervention.

For the second phase, often the counselor (and at times a spouse) will present the request to the alcoholic. The treatment program is explained to the alcoholic and the questions and objections are answered. The alcoholic may try to bargain around entering a formal program. When employers are supportive and with third-party payment being available, most legitimate concerns can be answered.

At times, it is desirable to accept the bargain *as long as it is put in writing.* For example, John may promise "I will quit on my own and not take a drink for one year." The interveners then respond, "Alright John, but if you do take a drink you will enter this treatment program the same day." Then all persons sign the agreement.

Rarely does an addicted person quit on their own (only approximately 5% and most of those are early-stage drinkers). In John's case, he is a late-stage drinker and will be in treatment within a month's time.

A few other points regarding the intervention process:

1. There are no set number of persons to be included in the process. Generally, around five to seven plus the counselor are present.
2. Generally, fairly early in the day is the best time. This alleviates the interveners from becoming unduly tense and prohibits the drinker from being intoxicated during the presentation (usually).
3. If a bargain is agreed on, the family needs to stay in therapy in the meantime.

4. Intervention is an emotionally expensive method of attempting to help an alcoholic. The counselor must make sure those who will be involved are able to successfully complete this task.
5. If the family is unavailable or otherwise unable to complete an intervention, then other alternatives must be examined.
6. When intervention is not an option, the family probably needs to be referred to Al-Anon so that their recovery may proceed. Then the appropriateness of intervention can be reassessed in a timely manner.
7. Intervention has a very high percentage of success in getting the alcoholic into treatment (in the 95% range). However, this is but the first step in the recovery program.

Components of Family Therapy

Outpatient

If for any reason the alcoholic cannot enter inpatient therapy (e.g. it is unavailable in the area in which he lives), then outpatient treatment is an important resource.

These are but a few of the restrictions for the family. The inpatient staff is limited in terms of what can be offered to families when the alcoholic is not in treatment. Thus, the family who is motivated to help will need to seek assistance elsewhere.

The options are not as limited as once was the case. The family can now seek assistance from a private practitioner, outpatient alcohol clinic or community mental health agency. Al-Anon always stands ready to assist the family.

The only caution to the family is this: if alcoholism at home is your problem, accept help only for this!

Education

No matter where treatment is sought, the family must be educated on the disease of alcoholism and how it has affected them. A component of this process is the bibliotherapy and the suggested reading list is provided at the end of this chapter.

Inpatient

Most of the family components of inpatient programs are

group related. Staffing shortages have dictated this approach as much as any other factor. Groups do allow the commonality and relating to each other's needs that family members often seek. This also allows dissemination of information and education to proceed. Some programs utilize some form of a weekly social event, planned by the inpatients and attended by the family. This facilitates learning to enjoy events, other people, and the family without alcohol.

Detrimental Family Attitudes

"Sobriety Will Cure All That Is Wrong." This belief is contrary to logic, yet is held by most family members. The family, especially those involved in interventions, must understand that sobriety is merely the beginning of months of intensive work and years of recovery.

"Everything That Is Wrong Is the Alcoholic's Fault." The most difficult aspect of providing treatment to the family is to help them understand their roles in the escalation of alcoholism.

Whenever a family system is dysfunctional, all members of the family have adopted some dysfunctional behaviors. The family members must be assisted to see this and instilled with a desire to grow and develop healthy attitudes and behaviors.

Treatment personnel need to determine what issues were unresolved in the marriage prior to the escalation of the drinking. This means adequate treatment, which combats this attitude.

"After All I've Done, Look at What has Happened." Treatment staffs have long confronted the alcoholic's pride and grandiosity, yet have remained silent when the spouse makes this statement. This is accurately labeled martyrdom and is the attitude most indicative of the spouse's own illness process. This attitude, if not dealt with decisively, will facilitate relapse.

At some point in treatment, the spouses need to receive couples' counseling to get all the troublesome issues expressed and explored.

Also, the attitude sometimes escalates into "I'm the one who has to keep him/her sober." This is so highly detrimental that it must be guarded against. Only the alcoholic alone can decide whether or not to take the first drink. Many factors can lead to a relapse and relapses need not be prolonged. The spouse's anxiety needs to be examined and treated.

"Now That She/He is Sober Everything Will Get Back to Normal." No such thing as normal exists in the alcoholic household. To expect that after all that has transpired the life-style that once existed will return is foolish. Neither spouse in the marriage is the same anymore. So, the couple must learn a lot about each other and, in most cases, must learn to love each other again.

"What if I don't Like Him/Her Now That Sobriety Has Been Achieved?" This is a major fear in the non-alcoholic spouse. If drinking has gone on for a significant amount of time, they may not really know each other. Family nights, AA parties, church activities and similar events are excellent ways for couples to get reacquainted with each other. Marital therapy is almost always necessary to restore the couple to a functioning relationship.

"I'm Here for You to Cure." This is an insidious attitude that often manifests itself through resistance to treatment assignments. The person's expectation is for the treatment staff to fix them rather than for the staff to challenge them. On the basis of the education and challenges placed in front of the individuals, they must work hard and change.

Therapy for the Elderly's Family

Any therapy for the elderly alcoholic by necessity includes the adult children, the grandchildren, spouse and siblings. This will pose a problem to a great many professionals. The family of the elderly is whomever that person has left. For alcoholics over the age of seventy, this is rarely a spouse. One of the stresses linked by all studies to reactive alcoholism is widowhood. Therefore, the reactive elderly alcoholic may be living with an adult child, a sibling or another relative. As their disease progresses, the surrounding people are affected just as any people around the alcoholic are affected.

The only time the family is completely unavailable is with the old–old category of people (over 74) when people have outlived all relatives. The other category of alcoholics without relatives is the chronic alcoholic who has long ago lost contact with the family. Aside from these two categories of people, assume the alcoholic has a family who needs therapy. Three kinds of therapy situations might occur. These are discussed in some detail next.

Spouse

The case history must ascertain, if possible, the quality of the relationship prior to the onset of the alcoholism.

This will assist the treatment team in knowing the needs of the spouse. Several factors influence whether the spouse will enter treatment or continue with therapy once they begin.

1. The length of the alcoholic's behavior and how the spouse has responded to the alcoholic.
2. Whether the spouse believes his/her involvement will make a difference.
3. Whether the spouse abuses alcohol or other chemicals.
4. The health and functional capacities of the spouse.
5. Whether the spouse accepts the treatment program philosophy (usually the disease concept).
6. The age of the spouse.
7. The length of the marriage.

The last two factors are most significant. If the couple has grown old together, the prognosis is good for both to recover. The fear and insecurity that the coalcoholic spouse endures must be treated in therapy.

Some of the emotional difficulties presented by spouses who have endured abuse and stress for several years may be beyond the capabilities of inpatient treatment staffs. Such a spouse may well need mental health and/or medical intervention beyond what can be given them. Such referrals need to proceed smoothly, with referral being made to a specific practitioner (never just to an agency).

When the marriage is an intergenerational one, the issues are somewhat different. Primarily, the pressure is on the older man, who may feel a need to perform at a high level for the younger woman. Major anxiety, sexual difficulties and financial concerns dominate. Usually, both spouses will report the same difficulties.

The overwhelming majority of intergenerational marriages are an older man and younger woman. As with all relationships, background information must be obtained. Has the relationship been intact for a long period of time? Generally, a difference of age in the twelve- to fifteen-year range qualifies this for an intergenerational marriage. Most of these marriages begin when the man is in his mid to late forties, and she is in her late twenties or early thirties. If the relationship has been good, then often the spouse enters and remains in therapy.

The other type of spouse is the product of remarriage. Careful assessment must determine how previous marriages ended and if alcoholism was involved. The level of comparison on an ex-spouse to the current spouse should also be evaluated.

Again, if extensive counseling is required for the spouse, a referral may be needed, since family counseling time is often limited for inpatient treatment staff. The primary concern must be to maximize the recovery potential for the troubled spouse.

Adult Children

The children of the elderly alcoholic can be involved in several spheres. First, the elderly person may live with an adult child and family. This is particularly true if the parent has been widowed.

If the parent is the father, issues can become bizarre as the disease progresses. The man may stay unkempt and may even make passes at the women in the house. Some cases even include indecent exposure, abusive language and stealing money to buy liquor. The in-law may take the stand that results in the father being treated.

When the parent is the mother, the issues are often lack of neatness, house accidents (such as leaving a burner on, falls, etc.), and being a financial burden. The woman is often "protected" longer by the adult children before the level of difficulty is admitted.

One of the major concerns in either situation is to treat the family dysfunction that often exists without the alcoholism. For the children to become caretaker and be in charge requires a high level of adjustment on both the parents and the child's part. Often, no one is available to advise and assist in this difficulty. Good information has been impossible to find for many.

When the parent is being cared for because of disability, then the burden is more difficult for both. The bibliotherapy for families list indicates a reliable source of information for both children and the parent.

When the adult child enters therapy they often fit right into the family group. Most are eager and involved. At times, their eagerness must be tempered with a conviction that they need help, also.

The second way the adult child becomes involved is as adjunct to both parents being in treatment. Often the initial call for program information is from a child who is concerned and willing to risk contact.

Again, assessment must reveal the extent of the impact the disease has had on the children. Then appropriate therapy should be rendered.

Siblings

As spouses outlive their partners, more are beginning to live with their siblings (also, often alone for whatever reason). Increasingly, this has been sisters who are close throughout life. Because of the lifetime closeness, the sibling may be the most protective of all family members, especially if the sibling has never encountered alcoholism previously.

Both sisters in this situation will require careful, gentle attention. The level of disability can often be reduced, and the two will often remain involved with the program throughout recovery.

Less common is to find two brothers living together late in life, yet this also occurs. One note of caution: both brothers may be involved in alcohol abuse to varying degrees. To attempt to treat one as the "family" and one as the "alcoholic" will be disastrous. Treatment staffs must be careful to pay close attention to this phenomenon and what one says about the other's alcohol intake.

Distant Relatives

More distant relatives, such as nephews, nieces and cousins, are also involved when alcoholism strikes someone who is in their care. The stickiest of situations arise when a distant relative is guardian of the estate or payee for the person's funds but is otherwise unwilling to be involved in the elderly person's life. Social service intervention will usually be resisted. At times, drinking behavior has been responsible for distancing. However, often the person is simply discharging "duty" and has no interest beyond.

When alcoholism is suspected, then the relative will often withhold funds, which can seriously endanger the elderly person. Whenever these persons can be included and taught, the better off all involved will be.

Outpatient Therapy

Quite frequently, a person enters outpatient therapy because the situation is so painful that it simply cannot be carried on as things are at the time. However, as the situation improves, the person will often drop out of treatment because things are the best they have been in years.

Mrs. J was such an example. After six therapy sessions on an outpatient basis by a gerontologist who specialized in alcohol, she came to realize that she was the classic coalcoholic. This was accomplished through education and bibliotherapy using general information and pamplets geared to a rural junior high education. What developed was enough ego strength that she was able to tell her son, who was in his twenties and who was also an alcoholic, that he simply had to leave home and develop a life on his own, which he did. She felt the most positive about herself that she had in years because of being able to finally clear up one of the situations at home that was causing her so much distress. When the son left, the husband's drinking decreased, the marriage improved and the client dropped out of therapy, citing "things are fine now, thank you."

Unfortunately, since the wife did not completely follow through on treatment and since the husband was still refusing treatment, predictably the improvement did not last long. The client had to be readmitted on an inpatient crisis unit and now will assume outpatient therapy once more.

This is not an uncommon problem in outpatient therapy. Professionals that contend that the crisis point is the best way to get a person into treatment are absolutely correct. However, if inpatient treatment is either not available or undesirable at the time, the crisis often wanes and so does the interest in therapy. Careful attention must be given by the professional in this setting in keeping the person involved in therapy by using both educational as well as directed therapeutic approaches.

Also necessary is to attempt to convince the individual early in therapy of how many sessions they will be required to keep in order to see an improvement that has a chance of lasting. Therapy in an outpatient setting has dual goals. The first goal is to treat the coalcoholic to alleviate their stress by understanding what's happened to them. The second goal is to get the person who is the alcoholic also into treatment. It should be stressed to the individual that they cannot do it for the other person, but that they have to do this for themselves.

Another note of caution is that they need to be informed that growth in their lives in breaking out of the games and the methods of the relationship that have caused pain and been dysfunctional quite often produces one of two results. The first and desired result is that the individual that comes into treatment grows, develops, changes, and becomes able to face life with or without the alcoholic. The desirable goal at that point is that the person that is doing the drinking will also want to grow and they will also come in for treatment. However, an equal possibility is that the person who is drinking may see the growth and development and may not want part of the marriage or the person any longer. An agenda that does not include information on those two points is likely to produce a dropout if the alcoholic does indeed resent the outside interference or the growth of his/her partner.

This is part of the sick game that an alcoholic will play to keep the spouse enslaved to the relationship and to the drinker. Even though life is miserable, particularly if the coalcoholic is a woman, at least she has a husband, usually a home, and some form of security. To ask her to risk that by getting well is indeed a tall request that cannot be taken lightly. The therapist who does not deal with that is likely to have a high dropout rate among the coalcoholics being treated and may never know why.

Family Dos and Don'ts

The following dos and don'ts were recommended by Muriel Zink in her book, *Ways to Live More Comfortably With Your Alcoholic.* *

---

*From Muriel Zink, *Ways To Live More Comfortably With Your Alcoholic.* © 1977. Courtesy of CompCare Publications, 2415 Annapolis Lane, Minneapolis, Minnesota 55441.

DO be honest with your spouse and yourself. Say what you mean and mean what you say. Alcoholism is the problem—not all the other issues you focus on.

DON'T play games and preach or lecture.

DO let the alcoholic's supply be visible, and be matter of fact about his or her need for it.

DON'T hide or dispose of liquor.

DO make your decision as to stay or go—and when your alcoholic is not drinking, tell your loved one of your plans and the "why" of them. One woman left her husband with the words, "I love you too much to sit around helplessly while you destroy yourself."

DON'T threaten to leave unless you intend to follow through.

DO explain the nature of the disease and the precautions to be taken.

DON'T try to pretend to children that nothing is wrong.

DO be open, reasonable and honest, accepting the illness as you would heart trouble, ulcers, etc.

DON'T try to hide the fact of your alcoholic's disease from others.

DO obtain and read literature provided by the National Council on Alcoholism, Alcoholics Anonymous, Al-Anon and other reputable sources; attend AA and Al-Anon meetings; talk with people who have experienced the joy of recovery.

DON'T listen to the prejudiced, judgmental "experts" who see alcoholism as a weakness of character.

DO remember that the progression of the disease has taken its toll on everyone concerned. The alcoholic has created a lifestyle which is centered around alcohol, and attitudes and habit patterns have been established which are difficult to alter. You, as well, have constructed a defense and denial structure which does not change easily.

DON'T expect that everything in your life will become perfect if and when your alcoholic stops drinking.

DO recognize your need for enlightened self-interest, for trust, for faith, and for the willingness to take responsibility for your own actions and attitudes.

DON'T depend on people or circumstances for your well-being or source of happiness.

DO remember that for those who avail themselves of help and treatment, the recovery rate is higher than for any other chronic progressive disease.

DON'T give up!

BIBLIOTHERAPY FOR FAMILIES

Drews, Toby Rice: *Getting them Sober*. New Jersey: Haven Books, 1980.

Maxwell, Ruth: *The Booze Battle*. New York: Ballantine Books, 1976.

Silverstone, Barbara; and Hyman, Helen Kandel: *You and Your Aging Parents*. New York: Pantheon Books, 1982.

Wegscheider, Sharon: *The Family Trap*. Minnesota: Nurturing Networks, 1976.

Zink, Muriel: *Ways to Live More Comfortably with Your Alcoholic*. Minneapolis: CompCare Publications, 1977.

SUGGESTED READINGS FOR PROFESSIONALS
WORKING WITH FAMILIES

Kinney, Jean; and Leaton, Gwen: *Loosening the Grip. A Handbook of Alcohol Information*. St. Louis: C. V. Mosby Company, 1978.

Maxwell, Ruth: *The Booze Battle*. New York: Ballantine Books, 1976.

Wegscheider, Sharon: *Another Chance: Hope and Health for the Alcoholic Family*. Palo Alto, California: Science and Behavior Books, Inc. 1981.

Chapter 11

SELF-HELP GROUPS
Alcoholism Recovery

SELF-help groups have arisen to facilitate recovery for specific groups of alcoholics and their families. The effectiveness of the groups is demonstrated by their continued growth in numbers and the outcomes of their efforts.

Alcoholics Anonymous

Historical

The prototype of recovery and group effectiveness for self-help groups, this fellowship has grown in geometric proportions since the group's inception in 1939 in Akron, Ohio. Alcoholics Anonymous (AA) is an evolution of people afflicted with alcoholism using a trial-and-error approach. Although one of the two founders of AA was Doctor Bob, the group was not founded as a science or as a professional organization. Rather, one alcoholic who was tempted to drink (Bill W.) sought out another and the fellowship was born. As the group grew to about 100 members in 1939, the members decided to compile their experiences in gaining sobriety. The result of this effort, written in past tense, is the book, *Alcoholics Anonymous* (also called the *Big* book). The group continued its growth in the Akron area until 1941 when AA received publicity in a national publication. Since that article appeared, the fellowship of AA has become a worldwide entity with over one million members.

General Information

Alcoholics Anonymous has two kinds of meetings. The first is the open meeting, which is literally for any interested individual who wishes to attend. This may be either a discussion group led by an AA member (usually not the same member on a regular basis), with the topic of discussion being chosen by a member or guest's questions, or there may be a guest speaker who is invited to address the meeting. The second type of meeting is the closed meeting. In the closed meeting, only members of AA attend. These meetings center on twelve-step work and specific issues pertaining to the recovering alcoholics in the group.

The philosophy of AA is found in the twelve steps and twelve traditions, which are listed below:

The Twelve Steps

1. We admitted we were powerless over alcohol—that our lives had become unmanageable.
2. Came to believe that a Power greater than ourselves could restore us to sanity.
3. Made a decision to turn our will and our lives over to the care of God *as we understood Him.*
4. Made a searching and fearless moral inventory of ourselves.
5. Admitted to God, to ourselves, and to another human being the exact nature of our wrongs.
6. Were entirely ready to have God remove all these defects of character.
7. Humbly asked Him to remove our shortcomings.
8. Made a list of all persons we had harmed and became willing to make amends to them all.
9. Made direct amends to such people wherever possible, except when to do so would injure them or others.
10. Continued to take personal inventory and when we were wrong promptly admitted it.
11. Sought through prayer and meditation to improve our conscious contact with God *as we understood Him*, praying only for knowledge of His will for us and the power to carry that out.

12. Having had a spiritual awakening as the result of these steps, we tried to carry this message to alcoholics and to practice these principles in all our affairs.

The Twelve Traditions

1. Our common welfare should come first; personal recovery depends upon AA unity.
2. For our group purpose there is but one ultimate authority— a loving God as He may express Himself in our group conscience. Our leaders are but trusted servants; they do not govern.
3. The only requirement for AA membership is a desire to stop drinking.
4. Each group should be autonomous except in matters affecting other groups or AA as a whole.
5. Each group has but one primary purpose—to carry its message to the alcoholic who still suffers.
6. An AA group ought never endorse, finance, or lend the AA name to any related facility or outside enterprise, lest problems of money, property and prestige divert us from our primary purpose.
7. Every AA group ought to be fully self-supporting, declining outside contributions.
8. Alcoholics Anonymous should remain forever non-professional. but our service centers may employ special workers.
9. AA, as such, ought never be organized; but we may create service boards or committees directly responsible to those they serve.
10. Alcoholics Anonymous has no opinion on outside issues; hence, the AA name ought never be drawn into public controversy.
11. Our public relations policy is based on attraction rather than promotion; we need always maintain personal anonymity at the level of press, radio, and films.
12. Anonymity is the spiritual foundation of our traditions, ever reminding us to place principles before personalities.

AA Alone

When AA was begun in 1939, no "scientific" or formal treatment programs existed. The AA method became a program as the trial-and-error approach became refined. Thus, much of the hardline approach of AA towards treatment is due to the school-of-hard-knocks approach. Although this attitude is not prevalent throughout AA, this attitude is expressed by some members on occasion. Part of the turf-guarding has been due to misconceptions of both AA and treatment program personnel. Neither has been really aware of what the other does. The results have usually been confusion, disillusionment and a ready excuse for the newly recovering alcoholic. This is most unfortunate, since the two are not competitive models.

The hallmark of AA and the reason for the phenomenal success of AA is the fellowship. For many, AA is the first attempt at contact with people after sobering up. The fellowship of AA is a handshake, a pat on the back, the offer of a cup of coffee. By virture of arriving at the meeting, the person is accepted and welcomed. The fellowship of AA allows the individual a positive range of people and behaviors to which to relate. The fellowship removes the question of where to spend leisure time, how to enjoy a social setting without alcohol, and family involvement. Friendships are often formed by the time a person attends two or three meetings. Then the alcoholic learns something important: alcoholics are more alike than different. This lesson makes working a twelve-step program, sponsorship, closed meetings, and reaching out to others possible.

The stories told by alcoholics have always been so similar in many key characteristics. These have been called defects of character, such as dishonesty, resentment and fear, to name a few.

The twelve-step program is a daily way of life. The program, when applied, teaches self-acceptance, growth, change and friendship. The program teaches the honesty on which interpersonal relationships must be based.

Because AA is open to all persons who are either problem drinkers or alcohol addicted, the appeal is tremendous. Alcoholics Anonymous has no formal organization or leadership, no professional therapy is rendered, no fees are required, members truly are anonymous, and the groups are available in virtually every area.

AA as Part of Professional Treatment

As the treatment approaches of alcoholism programs and mental health centers have been refined and developed, AA has been challenged. In areas where feuds have developed between some AA members and some treatment personnel, both programs have been devalued. For some reason, people have felt that their way is the only way. This mutually exclusive attitude prohibits the cooperation and mutual benefits of the approaches. The goal of both program approaches is the same: to produce sobriety that will result in lasting recovery for both the alcoholic and the family. To fail to cooperate is to make a feud more important than their purpose.

Professional treatment has several advantages as does AA. When the two groups work together, the best possible sobriety for the alcoholic results. While aftercare is important, AA provides this globally, and while the twelve-step program works, intensive education and inpatient treatment may be the beginning the alcoholic requires. Thus, the two can function together. In fact, every professional program introduces their patients to AA while in their program. To reduce this to feuding is inexcusable. Peer pressure can reduce such behavior immediately (and should).

Conclusion

Alcoholics Anonymous is "a complete or nearly complete philosophical approach to the process of daily living," and, "while not a form of treatment, AA has nonetheless significantly contributed to the ongoing sobriety of countless numbers of formerly hopeless alcoholics" (Forrest, 1978). These two statements are the bottom line on AA. To become involved in needless arguments and controversy involving the components of AA is ridiculous behavior.

Al-Anon

This is the family component of AA. The Al-Anon program fully embraces the twelve steps and twelve traditions as they are applied to the family, particularly spouses, parents and siblings. The Al-Anon program embodies fellowship and support. The spouse often seeks Al-Anon when all else has failed and help must be sought for the alcoholic. Gently and quickly, the group will teach the family of their personal need to recover *irregardless of what the alcoholic does in the future.*

Since Al-Anon is not under the restraints of time that professional programs experience, Al-Anon often becomes a haven for the suffering family. Often, the family's recovery enables the alcoholic to admit the need for help.

The recovery rate in Al-Anon is impressive and combines the twelve-step program with education and support. The similarities of stories among Al-Anon members is most startling to some. Yet, because of the similarities, the family's sanity is restored.

Surprisingly, Al-Anon is not perceived as a threat to treatment staffs as is AA. Thus, many of the aforementioned difficulties are not encounted.

Al-Anon enables the significant others to be part of the solution instead of part of the problem.

Ala-Teen

This is the AA program model for teenagers. As with Al-Anon, the teens are able to be heard and understood; to grow and change. The twelve steps are applied to themselves. As with Al-Anon, the Ala-Teen group permits a restoration of sanity for the most innocent victims of alcoholism—the children. Because the children are introduced to recovery, often the long-range effects of the parental alcoholism never develop. This is perhaps prevention at its highest form!

The meetings are often held in schools and churches. A function of guidance counselors is to determine who are in need of the Ala-Teen group and to see that the student gets there.

AA in the Gay Community

Statistically, the highest relapse rate among alcoholics belongs to this category. The highest suicide rate and dropout treatment rate also belongs to this category. Some studies report as many as

32 percent of all homosexuals are actively abusing alcohol. The major stress involved against the gay community contributes to this addiction process. Further, the gay bar is the hub of social activities with the least stress and aggravation. The bar scene is one of the major reasons for the high relapse rate. Alcoholics Anonymous now has over 300 gay groups throughout the United States. Likewise, groups called Alcoholics Together (AT) and Women for Sobriety have also been formed and are growing quickly both in numbers and in effectiveness.

AA for Women

Many women have discovered some of the stresses that face them are different than those that face men. Thus, closed AA meetings of women only have grown more popular. Some of these stresses include menopause, motherhood, keeping a house, caring for a spouse, and career-oriented pressures. The burden of entertaining is often on the wife. All of these unique needs are dealt with in addition to others.

Chapter 12

NUTRITION AND EXERCISE

Rebuilding the Body

NUTRITION and exercise are vital components in all age groups for building sobriety following years of drinking behavior. This is vital for the elderly more than any other age group.

The loss of reserve capacity in the elderly requires careful attention to be given to helping the elderly alcoholic realize the proteins, vitamins, and minerals that the body requires are lost during drinking. Attending to this during the treatment program itself is important. In the time period after discharge and completing a treatment program, the elderly must follow a program of nutrition and exercise or face relapse.

Ideally, every alcoholic that comes in for treatment in this age group will have the financial resources to buy the foods, vitamins and minerals that the body requires in rebuilding itself. The reality of this is much different. For the therapist treating an alcoholic in this age group, considerable education and attention must be given these people with regard to nutrition. For the therapist, this may mean helping to fill out a food stamp application and having a volunteer from the program accompany the elderly person to a food stamp office. This may be having the dietitian, if it's a hospital-based program, lecture to these individuals in this age group, particularly on how to get the basic food requirements for the least amount of money. For the elderly alcoholic, if this area is not stressed and taught thoroughly during treatment, relapse is fairly well guaranteed. Many treatment programs stress the need for vitamins and minerals during the hospitalization itself. This is also vital once the alcoholic returns to the home environment.

While research shows that it takes up to seven years of vitamin deprivation for a healthy adult to show signs of a vitamin deficiency, this is not the case in the elderly alcoholic. Figure 12-1 shows the essential ingredients for a multipurpose vitamin and mineral supplement. Vitamins A and D, which are stored in the liver and other body organs, are rapidly destroyed by alcohol abuse. The vitamins C and B complex, which are so vital in the elderly for fighting infections, are also severely depleted during the drinking process. Also common in the elderly alcoholic during the initial attempted sobriety is a craving for sweets, particularly chocolate, sweet rolls with frosting, and some other kinds of very sweet foods. If the treatment staff notices a person craving this type of food, careful attention needs to be given to the blood sugar level of the individual and whether or not the individual is self-treating hypoglycemia by eating the sweets. Since metabolism also decreases and also very frequently physical activity decreases, body fats can build up at a high rate. This is also a problem in treatment programs for those who do not need to gain weight, who notice the return of appetite perhaps for the first time in years and tend to overeat during the treatment program and not get the exercise needed, thus gaining weight rapidly. Figure 12-1 shows the vitamins and minerals that should be taken at least six months following sobriety. Several brand name companies market these vitamin/mineral combinations at affordable prices.

Insurance tables indicate that a 55–75-year-old average man of average build should consume approximately, 2,200 calories a day. The average size/average build woman in the same age group should consume in the neighborhood of 1,600 calories a day. This may need to be adjusted upwards or downwards contingent upon whether the individual is overweight or underweight coming into treatment. Also, careful attention needs to be given to whether this person ever had a weight problem in the past, either gaining or losing weight rapidly.

VITAMIN MINERAL SUPPLEMENT

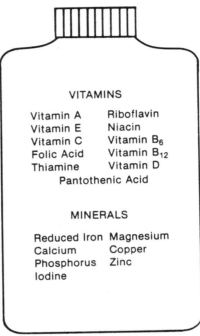

VITAMINS

Vitamin A	Riboflavin
Vitamin E	Niacin
Vitamin C	Vitamin B_6
Folic Acid	Vitamin B_{12}
Thiamine	Vitamin D
Pantothenic Acid	

MINERALS

Reduced Iron	Magnesium
Calcium	Copper
Phosphorus	Zinc
Iodine	

Figure 12-1. Any multipurpose vitamin/mineral supplement for rebuilding a healthy body should utilize these components.

Other important considerations in terms of diet are whether or not there are indications of hardening of the arteries or arteriosclerosis, heart condition, or high blood pressure in the past medical history. If there are any of these conditions, then a dietitian needs to work very carefully to teach the person what they can have to eat and the kinds of food they should avoid for better health. Menu suggestions and guidelines are most helpful.

Since the person is being treated for drug addiction, the less routine medications these people are on, the better the recovery prognosis. For example, if an individual's high blood pressure can be treated by the person using a salt substitute, getting more exercise and eating a good basic diet, this is preferable to placing the person on a medication, thus making the person chemically dependent once again. A thorough dietary history will often indicate the cause for high blood pressure, and medication is not required.

Also of concern in this age bracket is the condition of the teeth and/or dentures. Obviously, any individual who is missing most of their teeth is going to have some digestive problems since any food that is consumed cannot adequately be chewed up, hampering the digestive process. Some of the meat products that the person might otherwise be able to eat are eliminated from the diet because the meat cannot be chewed up at all. Medicaid and Medicare will help with the price of dentures if a physician certifies that their physical health will be improved as a result of having teeth. Certainly, attempting to sit down and eat a hamburger with no teeth or any other number of foods would be most difficult if a person cannot take a bite of the food and chew it up adequately.

Some basic home cooking hints might be very appropriate for a widowed male or for those in retirement communities who do not fix their food.

Basic Diet

The four basic food groups must be represented in the daily diet. These are the meat group, the dairy food group, the fruits and vegetables group, and the bread and cereal group. An outline of an exchange diet such as the one that the American Diabetes Association gives to diabetics or the one that Upjohn gives to some of their persons on home health care can be quite useful in teaching persons where the food falls in the various food groups.*

Meats
Meat (beef, lamb, pork, liver) slice 3″ × 2″ × 1/2″ or approximately 3 oz. cooked
Poultry (chicken, duck, turkey) 3-4 oz. cooked

---

*Diet lists were compiled by author from diet lists of American Diabetes Association, U.S. Public Health Service, the Upjohn Company, and a personal physician's suggested diet.

Frankfurter—1 dinner size or 2 regular
Codfish, halibut, mullett, sole, etc. (4 oz. cooked)
Salmon, tuna, crab, lobster—1/4 cup
Oysters, shrimps, clams (5-6)
Sardines (3)
Cheese—Cheddar, American or Swiss—1 oz.
Cottage cheese—1/4 cup
Egg—1
Peanut butter—1 tbsp. (limit this to one serving daily)

Milk

Milk, whole, 1 cup
Milk, evaporated, 1/2 cup
Milk, powered, 1/4 cup
Milk, skim, 1 cup
Buttermilk, 1 cup
Yogurt, 1/2 cup

Breads

Bread (white, wheat or grain) 1 slice
Biscuit roll, 1 (2″ in diameter)
Muffin, 1 (2″ in diameter)
Cornbread, 1 1/2″ cube
Flour - 2 1/2 tbsp.
Cereal, cooked (1/2 cup) such as cream of wheat
Cereal, dry (puffed or flakes) 3/4 cup
Rice, 1/2 cup, cooked
Grits, 1/2 cup, cooked
Spaghetti, macaroni, noodles, 1/2 cup cooked
Crackers, graham (2)
Crackers, oyster (20 or 1/2 cup)
Crackers, saltines (5)
Crackers, round (8)
Sponge cake (plain) 1 1/2″ cube
Ice cream—1/2 cup
Vegetables (in bread category)
　　Beans (lima, navy) 1/2 cup, cooked
　　Peas (split or green) 1/2 cup, cooked
　　Baked beans—1/4 cup
　　Corn—1/3 cup

Parsnips—2/3 cup
Potatoes, sweet—1/4 cup
Potatoes, white—baked or boiled 1 (2″ diameter)
Potatoes, white—mashed, 1/2 cup

Group I. Eat all of this list desired if *uncooked. If cooked,* then eat 1 cup as 1 serving.

Asparagus	Cauliflower	Eggplant
Broccoli	Celery	Escarole
Brussell sprouts	Chicory	
Cabbage	Cucumber	
Chard	Mushrooms	Sauerkraut
Collards	Okra	Stringbeans
Dandelion	Parsley	Squash, summer
Kale	Peppers (green or red)	Tomatoes
Mustard	Radishes	Water cress
Poke	Romaine	Sprouts, bean
Spinach	Rhubarb	Turnips
Lettuce		

Group II. 1 serving = 1/2 cup. 1 cup of Group I vegetables may be substituted for Group II vegetables.

Beets	Onions	Pumpkin	Squash, winter
Carrots	Peas	Rutabagas	Turnips

Fruits

Apple—1 small	Grapes, 12
Applesauce, 1/2 cup	Grape juice, 1/4 cup
Apricots, fresh, 2 medium	Honeydew melon, 1/8
Apricots, dried, 4 halves	Mango
Berries, 1 cup	Orange, 1
blackberries	Orange juice, 1/2 cup
raspberries	Papaya, 1/3 medium
strawberries	Peach, 1 medium
Blueberries, 2/3 cup	Pears, 1
Cantaloupe. 1/4	Plums, 2
Cherries, 10 large	Prunes, dried 2
Dates, 2	Prune juice, 1/4 cup
Figs, fresh, 1 large	Raisins, 2 tbsps.
Figs, dried, 1 large	Tangerine, 1
Grapefruit, 1/2	Watermelon, 1 cup
Grapefruit juice, 1/2 cup	Pineapple, 1/2 cup

Fats

Butter or margarine, 1 tsp.
Bacon, crisp, 1 slice
Cream, 2 tbsps.
  light
  sour
  sweet
  whipped
Cream cheese, 1 tbsp.

French dressing, 1 tbsp.
Mayonnaise, 1 tsp.
Oil or lard, 1 tsp.
Nuts, 1 oz.
Olives, 5
Avocado, 1/8
Cream, heavy, 1 tbsp.

Unlimited Foods

Coffee
Tea
Broth
Bouillon
Lemon
Gelatin (unsweet)
Cranberries (unsweet)

Pickles
Saccharin
Pepper
Spices
Seasonings
Low-calorie soft drinks
Mustard (dry)

Tips to Remember

Endless varieties of salads can be made utilizing the vegetables in Groups I and II. Also, the taste will vary when meat (such as tuna and chicken) and salad dressings are added.

Fruit solids should be eaten rather than the juice, since a fruit eaten whole takes two hours to digest, while the fruit juice lasts for only thirty minutes.

Utilize farmer's markets, vegetable stands, pick your own vegetables and fruit stands rather than the supermarket for the best buys on these items. If a person lives in a rural area, some fruits and vegetables can be either picked fresh from the field by the individual or bought at a vegetable stand.

Clean and fix vegetables for a several day period at the same time and store in a vegetable crisper to eliminate the bother of cleaning them each time they are desired.

Broil, bake, charcoal or grill meats often, as this is most healthy method of cooking and gains maximum benefits from the food.

When buying canned fruits try to buy those packed in "natural juice," instead of syrup, as this is preferable, especially for the overweight person.

Do *not* eliminate all fats from the diet. Research indicates hormone levels are regulated in part by fat in the diet. These are essential to good health in every age bracket.

Although the diet or sugar-free drinks can be consumed freely, pay some heed to amount of caffeine in cola, root beer, and similar sodas.

Snack on celery, carrots, squash, popcorn, and avoid sweet foods.

Helpful Cooking Hints

Occasionally, combine vegetables and meat in the form of stews, pot roast with potatoes and carrots, chicken and rice casserole.

Combine leftovers when possible. Meats can be added to a sauce with rice or noodles to make a delicious, one dish type meal.

Cream or grind leftover meats (often an electric mixer has a grinder function) and add to any of the creamed soups for an inexpensive sauce.

Garnish ordinary-looking foods with something that is eye catching, such as a slice of pepper, a pickle, a piece of parsley, or a leaf of lettuce.

Food tastes (especially important for weight-loss programs) can be changed by using Worcestershire sauce, soy sauce, spices, fruit juices and mixes prepared and sold at supermarkets. Eating a limited diet need not be bland. Fixed incomes are much more bearable when variety can be introduced into the diet.

Other important issues in the nutrition realm include the need for drinking water every day. If drinking water from the tap is not tasty, try boiling it for freshness. Also, supermarkets now sell mineral or spring water at a nominal cost. Many nutritional difficulties that plague the elderly are a result of lack of water consumption. Two of the major maladies of poor digestion and constipation could be eliminated simply by drinking a quart of water daily. This also eliminates tendency of kidneys and urinary tract problems in the elderly woman. This is of particular concern if the drinking history has been severe.

Exercise

The second aspect of importance to overall well-being is that of exercise. Ideally, each elderly person has an exercise program that was developed early in life and followed into the retirement years. The popular sterotype of the elderly is that of the little old people out playing shuffleboard in a retirement center shuffleboard court. Doubtless, after age sixty-five, all persons are required to know how to play shuffleboard. Certainly, this is not the case. The elderly alcoholic may need assistance in restructuring their leisure activities, but the activities of the past can still be enjoyed in the older years.

Leisure activities such as bicycling, swimming, tennis, softball, table tennis, billiards and similar activities can be enjoyed throughout life with minor modifications in a team sport such as softball. Many elderly alcoholics have returned to sports such as golf with renewed enthusiasm and interest. Elderly persons who belong to activity centers or country clubs are involved in multiple activities. These activities can easily be enjoyed by most elderly persons throughout their sixties and seventies. For the elderly who are restricted in their activities by arthritis, injury, or some serious illness, walking is the exercise of choice. Walking is a healthy activity and is available to most people. By walking, each of the body systems are strengthened. One researcher even hypothesized that one reason women outlive men is the amount of walking required in shopping, housekeeping, child rearing (including the grandchildren) and other daily activities.

Persons who have weight problems, arthritis, or have suffered a fracture can benefit tremendously by exercise such as toe touches, stretching, sit-ups, and specific activities suggested by the physician (see Figures 12-2 and 12-3). These activities can be enjoyed throughout a person's life span.

Successful treatment programs build some exercise periods into a daily program. The attitude of the person towards the daily activities will be a good indicator of how persons will care for themselves in the future.

The benefits of exercise are well known and documented. However, the person who was addicted to one or more substances may not be excited about doing these things that rebuild the body. If the staff and program alumni are excited about the exercise times, this attitude can be imparted to the newly recovering person.

Also, fun kinds of activities can be done, including dancercise (get the older members to demonstrate the "oldie" dances).

EXERCISE EDDIE: JOINT ROTATIONS

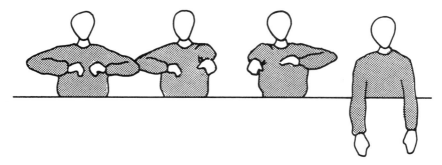

Figure 12-2. Joint rotation exercises insure continued use of joints (in the absence of disease). These can be done anywhere.

EXERCISE EDDIE: SEMI-KNEE BENDS

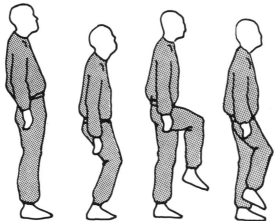

Figure 12-3. Semi-knee bends are designed to keep legs, thighs, and lower torso firm.

By utilizing sensible diet and moderate exercise, a good measure of physical well-being can be reestablished. Thus, the positive attitude towards self and others and a sense of controlling one's own life will produce new self-confidence for solving life's everyday problems.

Exercise Eddie

Basic exercises are required for muscle tone (see Figures 12-4–12-10). Exercise Eddie demonstrates each of these exercise. Of primary concern is getting the benefits of the exercise without risking injury. Thus, as shown in Figures 12-4 and 12-6, a wall can be used for support.

One of the advantages of exercise is the slowing of some age-related difficulties. Other signs of aging occur regardless (see Figure 12-11).

EXERCISE EDDIE: WALL PUSH-UPS

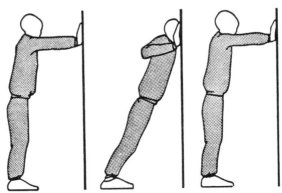

Figure 12-4. This exercise allows the upper body the benefits of push-ups without straining the back.

**EXERCISE EDDIE:
SIT-UPS UTILIZING BACK SUPPORTS**

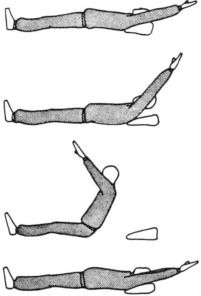

Figure 12-5. Sit-ups using a back support enable the light exercise to attain stomach tone without strain to the back.

**EXERCISE EDDIE:
KNEE BENDS UTILIZING WALL FOR SUPPORT**

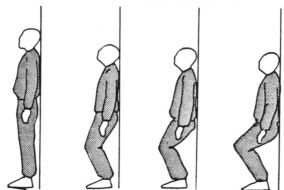

Figure 12-6. Unless one is in good physical condition, a wall can be utilized to prohibit falls and to reduce chances of injury.

EXERCISE EDDIE: LEG LIFTS

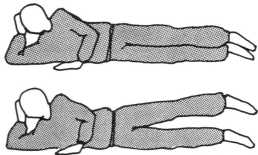

Figure 12-7. Leg lifts help tone muscles that are not utilized much of the time.

EXERCISE EDDIE: TOE TOUCHES

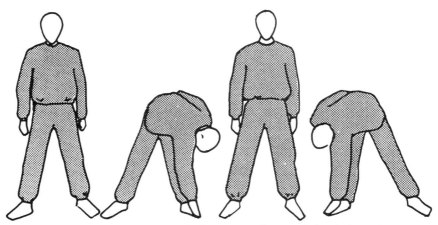

Figure 12-8. Toe touches provide for an excellent and simple torso toner.

EXERCISE EDDIE: NECK ROTATIONS

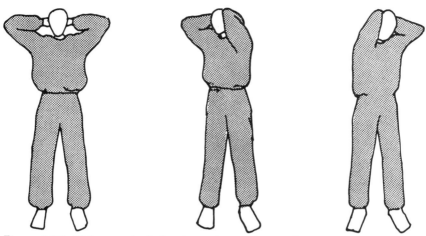

Figure 12-9. This exercise helps strengthen and tone the neck and upper back muscles and should precede most active sports and all weight-lifting programs.

EXERCISE EDDIE: ARM STRENGTHENING EXERCISES

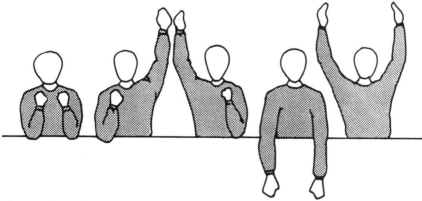

Figure 12-10. These are optional due to the frequency with which these muscles are utilized and can be included easily in all exercise programs.

EXERCISE EDDIE: PHYSICAL CHANGES AFTER 55

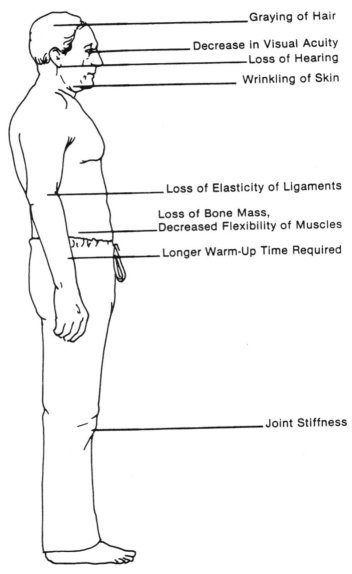

Graying of Hair

Decrease in Visual Acuity

Loss of Hearing

Wrinkling of Skin

Loss of Elasticity of Ligaments

Loss of Bone Mass, Decreased Flexibility of Muscles

Longer Warm-Up Time Required

Joint Stiffness

Figure 12-11. Exercise Eddie demonstrates the various changes that all elderly persons undergo after age 55. These changes do occur in varying degrees based on nutrition, exercise, and medical condition.

Exercise Tips

1. Consult a physician prior to beginning an exercise program. The physician can advise which activities will enhance the person's physical condition without aggravating chronic health problems.
2. Always wait approximately two hours after eating before engaging in more active exercise (such as tennis, jogging and golf).
3. Utilize (at least twice per week) activities that stimulate the heart. Such exercises include walking, bicycling, swimming and tennis.
4. Begin all exercise periods of strenuous activity by warming up. Good warm-up exercises include toe touches, stretching, sit-ups and windmills.
5. Likewise, end exercise periods by tapering off exercises. Cooling off periods should be in the same approximate temperature as the exercise to facilitate the body's returning to normal.
6. Older persons should not drink any form of alcoholic beverage while exercising (including a beer while mowing the yard), as the ethanol will act to dehydrate the body. This process is a leading cause of sun sickness and heat stroke in the elderly.
7. Drink only lukewarm–cool water at the peak of exercise periods, as this maximizes the body's utilization of the fluid. One of the available athlete drinks can be used if preferred.
8. The level of exercise should be maintained at a comfortable level. Chosen exercise should be enjoyable and invigorating.
9. Wear the appropriate clothing and shoes according to the activity. Dressing appropriately prevents accidents and injuries (and costs less than injury).
10. Exercise and activities are the best way to enjoy the company of others. Exercise will not only tone muscles and improve circulation but will also facilitate good digestion, weight control, bowel function and sleep patterns.

Chapter 13

CLERGYMAN'S GUIDE

Spirituality

DURING a group discussion one afternoon in a well-known treatment program, a question was raised for the counselor by one of the group members. The question was, How can I go about achieving spirituality? The therapist responded with a question, How is it that God will keep you from taking a drink? Alcoholics Anonymous, every church group, every religion as a whole, talks about how God helps us. If you want to take a drink, how can you avoid taking it and how will God help you avoid taking it?

The group was composed so that they have approximately twelve members. Six had achieved sobriety through Alcoholics Anonymous at some point, two of them were staunchly AA members and could tell you virtually every component of the AA program from heart, three had expressed a desire to return to churches that had in the past supported them and trained them, and three weren't sure what they would do to recover. Of the twelve people present in that group, no one was able to answer the question, How will God help you avoid taking a drink?

When the therapist explained the process of changing the inner person, of taking out of one's life a problem and replacing it with something wholesome and complete, they nodded and realized for the first time that God could be practical and could be real.

The book *Your God is Too Small*, by J. B. Phillips, has been a best-seller for many years. After extensive years of counseling alcoholics, therapists have become convinced that the problem is not that their God is too small, but that the problem is their God is not real. The difference in the two is astounding.

Many alcoholics, as well as the public at large, have the same view of God as adults that they had as small children—a view that says that God is a little, gray-bearded man that you call upon when you are in trouble and, being a nice old person, he will come down and help you. Some see this God as a "rocking chair God" who sits with a white beard and staff and legislates morality that people couldn't possibly fulfill. Others see God as a grade teacher as it were, someone who dashes about keeping track of everyone's faults and merits, so that on the day of judgment they can be balanced out to see who wins. Still another view of God is that of the cosmic bellhop; when in doubt, ring him up, when not, don't. Most people, after extensive years of discussing this with them, fall into those categories. God, as a personal father, is very troubling to someone who did not have a good relationship with their own father, so that to use an analogy of God as a caring father immediately dooms a person to have doubts and fears and negative attitudes.

Organized religion has not helped a great many persons in this process either. The failures of churches to produce changed lives and insure sobriety is more indicative of a problem within the church than for the alcoholic. Clergymen (whether discussing priests, rabbis, ministers, pastors, chaplains, or other church leaders) have as a group been unable to understand the complexity of alcoholism and all the forms of life change that are required to bring about a lasting sobriety in an individual.

Alcoholics Anonymous is a spiritual program that discusses spiritual growth and development in the life of an alcoholic to maintain sobriety. Further, the twelve steps states that if a person does not give this away, they cannot keep it for themselves. Anyone involved in a church on an active, daily basis will recognize the wisdom of such an approach and the completeness of such an approach. Alcoholics Anonymous differentiates between dry (i.e. just simply not drinking) and sober, which means that the person has a changed life—a life that is full and complete without alcohol. Certainly, any clergyman would wish to seek out an alcoholic and impart to them a sense of completeness and a sense of relationship with God that circumvents the sin, the feelings of guilt, the feelings of worthlessness, the feelings of hopelessness, and the feelings of alienation that alcoholics as a whole experience.

Many factors go into the lack of clergy effectiveness with alcoholism in general within their congregations. Part of this problem has been alcoholism in one's own family that has never been resolved. Since the clergy are also human beings, such unresolved issues will render them ineffective in dealing with that particular individual within their congregation. However, clergymen still need to understand alcoholism, and if this is a problem for them, they must overcome it.

Secondly, the clergymen have not understood alcoholism and what goes into building a spiritual, solid sobriety. Many have undertaken to provide a conversion experience to bring the alcoholic out of the feelings of worthlessness and into a fellowship within the congregation. However, that's been the end of it. A conversion experience must be the turning point; it must be the beginning. This does not involve a one-time experience that will always, for the rest of the person's life, deal with the problems in their life.

In fact, generally, a conversion experience, if the person really attempts to live the committments that they have made, produces a set of new problems and concerns as well. How tragic it has been for clergy to "convert" someone and tell them that now their alcoholism is resolved, only to have the person drink again. *This must be guarded against.*

Thirdly, the clergy, as a whole, has not understood what the Bible has to say regarding alcoholism and alcohol abuse. Alcoholism is not a problem common to this century or this time or, for that matter, to this culture. From the earliest Old Testament times throughout the New Testament, warnings were given against drunkenness and against abuse. The reason for these cautions was because alcohol abuse was a problem then as it is now. Proverbs 23:29–35 read like this:

> Who has woe? Who has sorrow? Who has strife? Who has complaining? Who has wounds without cause? Who has redness of eyes? Those who tarry long over wine, those who go to try mixed wine.

Do not look at wine when it is red, when it sparkles in the cup and goes down smoothly. At the last it bites like a serpent, and stings like an adder. Your eyes see strange things and your mind utters perverse things. You will be like one who lies down in the midst of the sea, like one who lies on top of a mask, 'they struck me' you will say, but 'I was not hurt, they beat me, but I did not feel it, when shall I awake? I will go seek another drink.'

This verse discusses delerium tremens, addiction, and the person who strives after nothing more than their next drink. This is the essence of alcoholism. To work with alcohol clients within a congregation is to be consistent with the Scriptures, and the clergy needs to begin to understand this. As with any other life-dominating problem, the whole life has to be restructured. The clergy is an important part of this team to do this.

Fourthly, the clergy has not understood that treatment programs and Alcoholics Anonymous are not mutually exclusive approaches to utilizing a church in the recovery process. There has been far too much turf guarding, far too much exclusiveness within all three factions, instead of a teamwork approach, whereby the clergy works with alcoholism treatment professionals and Alcoholics Anonymous members. In some of the major denominations, Alcoholics Anonymous meetings are actually held at the buildings of various churches throughout a community, and, thus, the clergymen involved have become consistently resourceful and knowledgeable in dealing with persons who suffer from alcoholism.

Fifthly, some clergy have seen themselves in somewhat of a bind because the Scriptures speak against drunkenness and speak against overindulgence in alcohol at will (or through loss of control) and, yet, in many other occasions sanction the use of wine. At the wedding feast, during the communion service and during the Agape dinners that were part of the early church, wine was used by members. Some of the arguments about this have been rather amusing. For example, some denominations have taught that any use of alcoholic beverage in this culture is wrong; that they had to use it in the early church only because water was not available. However, a careful review of John 4 will indicate that this argument is ridiculous. It certainly was not a drink of wine that Jesus asked for when He spoke to the woman drawing water from the well in that passage of Scriptures and many others like it. Also, in I Timothy 5:23, where Paul writing the young minister Timothy states, "No longer use only water, but use a little wine because of your stomach and frequent illnesses." This young minister on the basis of example and out of concern for his appearance for the church had drunk only water, which means that water was abundantly available even in that time. Certainly, a little alcohol has some medicinal values. The statistics bear this out. Those who drink moderately will outlive those who abstain, which debunks the teaching that if you abstain you will live longer and thereby glorify God. Statistically, this is not true; scripturally, it is not taught.

Another part of this dilemma for the clergy is the fact that Jesus' first miracle involved wine. This miracle took place at a wedding feast where Jesus turned barrels of water into wine. Of course, the fruit of the vine is a God-instituted part of a communion service in every Christian denomination in the world. However, fruit of the vine includes grape juice, just as well as grape wine, and a recovering alcoholic should be taken into consideration and should not be excluded from communion on the basis of trying to abstain from alcohol-containing beverages.

Clergy need to come to understand that the teachings of the Bible concerning wine and strong drink teach against overindulgence on anything that might render a person ineffective before God. Certainly, an alcoholic (a person who is not able to control the future of their lives once they take a drink) must begin to overcome what Jay Adams has referred to in his writings as a life-dominating sin. Certainly, anyone who turns to God for help, regardless of the condition of their life, will receive it. To teach anything else is to teach doctrines or beliefs that are totally erroneous in God's view. While the newly sober alcoholic is very easy to "convert," they bring a series of problems and a series of life-dominating attitudes and beliefs that have to change and have to be dealt with one at a time over several months. When the Christian church utilizes this approach, either in conjunction with other approaches or by itself, satisfying and complete change have occurred.

Sixthly, the clergy must come to understand that recovery from any addiction is a process, whether that be addiction to alcohol, drugs, nicotine, caffeine, or any other substance that people use to extremes. It is not a one for all, all for one kind of experience. The clergy must further understand that recovery is not just simply abstaining from a behavior that causes a significant number of problems in one's life. In Luke 11:24, the warning against this approach is given. It reads, "When an evil spirit comes out of a man, it goes through other places seeking rest and does not find it." Then it says, "I will return to the house I left." When it arrives, it finds the house swept clean and put in order. Then it goes and takes seven other spirits more wicked than itself and they go in and live there, and the final condition of that man is worse than the first.

To not stress the fundamental process of filling one's life up, once put in order, with things that are fulfilling and lasting and valuable to that human's existence is to set that person up for relapse. Churches and organized religions as a whole have done this to alcoholics more than any other group, including employers, family, friends, and other pursuits. The tragedy of this should not escape us.

An alcoholic who achieves some period of sobriety and pursues that sobriety and then loses it is much harder to reach a second time around and try to pull back into any kind of an approach to help this individual. The clergy must understand that alcoholism affects every area of someone's life as does any addiction. And that, while it is an indication that the person is not spiritually strong, is also an indication that they are not emotionally or physically strong either.

Seventh, the clergy has made a mistake in that, as a whole, they have not made God real to the people who attend their congregations. There is a difference between defining God for someone and sharing a relationship with God with someone. Although, at first glance this might seem to be the same thing, they are not. Most clergy are taught early in their ministries how to quote Scriptures about God's love, God's faithfulness, and all the good qualities that God has that is meant to encourage someone and yet leave someone wondering how to take those qualities of God for their own.

In a relationship with God, the individual is sharing in these qualities of God and can teach the person with them how to imitate this kind of relationship. Certainly, the scope of God presented in the Bible and in most religions is awesome, is frightening, and is mysterious. But love is that way, goodness is that way, the birth of a child is a wonder such as that, and people learn how to take advantage of enjoying those things without necessarily understanding every bit of it. The process is defined as "putting off the old self, and putting on the new self," which is documented in Colossians 3:1-17, Ephesians 5:18, and I Timothy 6:17.

A relationship with God is practical, specific, and oriented towards things to fulfill a human being and reach out to the people around them. Alcoholics Anonymous has produced this for hundreds of thousands of persons who have been unable to find it anywhere else. Treatment programs have produced and taught this. Yet, many church members have not been able to teach this kind of relationship.

Eighth, a relationship with God can be experienced. It has components that are definable, meaningful and which can be pursued. When the relationship is pursued and developed and grows, it produces a strong inner person that can deal with temptations and the pains and the consequences of a past life that no longer dominates the individual.

Again, clergy have, at times, set up alcoholics by failing to tell them that conversion will produce in them a change, which means that the old life will be totally and completely gone. And while spiritually this is the case in terms of the inner individual, this is not always the case in terms of the consequences brought on by an individual's actions prior to becoming involved with the church. This disciplined style of life includes many definable areas, and each must be discussed with the individual.

First, it produces a changed spiritual life. The person through conversion in Christ becomes a new creation. Buddhism, Hinduism, Judaism, and other religious groups have similar teachings. Problems still occur, life still has disappointments and pain; but the individual's approach changes. The attitude of enduring and overcoming by calling on a Power greater than self transcends the pain each will experience during life.

Secondly, new behaviors and attitudes do replace the old, habitual response of taking a drink. Honesty and ability to face one's self replaces lying and denying problems. Caring for others and serving their needs replaces resentments and bitterness. Contentment with one's place in life replaces envy and blind ambition. Growth in the person's life replaces stagnation, complacency and laziness. Relationships become meaningful and lasting instead of transitory.

Scriptural Guides

Somehow, the attitude has evolved that the concerns facing alcoholics/coalcoholics are somehow different than all other congregational members. Thus, when sought out for help, some clergymen have become unsure how to proceed.

The following is a Scriptural guide to the major causes of relapse in the alcoholic. As always, the Scriptures are practical, specific and timely. This guide does not purport to be exhaustive but to be an easy reference.

All Scriptures are from the New International Version of the New Testament (NIV) unless otherwise noted. (Zondervan, 1974). The NIV is the most accurate of the so-called modern translations and can be understood by anyone with basic reading skills. Although some denominations have vehemently denounced all post-King James translations, the emerging belief is that Bible study and guidance should be sought from a version that is easily understood. Many alcoholics encouraged to use the NIV have expressed surprise and pleasure at how easily they understood the Bible (for the first time!), and such should be the goal.

Complacency
"Whatever you do, work at it with all your heart."
(Colossians 4:23–25)

Grandiosity
"Do not think of yourself more highly than you ought, but rather think of yourself with sober judgment. . . ."
(Romans 12:3)

Emotionally Withdrawn
"Make room for us in your hearts."
(2 Corinthians 7:2)

"We are not withholding our affection from you, but you are withholding yours from us. . . ."

(2 Corinthians 6:11-13)

Ingratitude

"But if anyone does not have them, he is nearsighted and blind, and has forgotten that he has been cleansed from his past sins."

(2 Peter 1:8-9)

"Nor should there be obscenity, foolish talk or coarse joking, which are out of place, but rather thanksgiving."

(Ephesians 5:4)

Dishonesty

"Therefore, each of you must put off falsehood and speak truthfully to his neighbor, for we are all members of one body."

(Ephesians 4:25)

Euphoria

"Give and it will be given you. A good measure, pressed down, shaken together and running over, will be poured into your lap. . . ."

(Luke 6:38)

Forgiveness

"Be kind and compassionate to one another, forgiving each other just as God in Christ forgave you."

(Ephesians 4:32)

Service

"Do unto others as you would have them do unto you."

(Luke 6:31)

"Once you know these things, you will be blessed, if you do them."

(John 13:17)

Fear

"Do not let your hearts be troubled. Trust in God, trust also in me."

(John 14:1)

Self-Pity

"Finally, brothers, whatever is true, whatever is noble, whatever is right, whatever is pure, whatever is lovely, whatever is admirable—if anything is excellent or praiseworthy—think about such things."

(Philippians 4:8-9)

Unrealistic Goals

"But you man of God, shun all this and aim at righteousness, godliness, faith, love, steadfastness, gentleness."

(I Timothy 6:11)

Pride

"Therefore let anyone who thinks he stands take heed lest he falls."

(I Corinthians 10:12)

Mood-Altering Chemicals

"So then, do not be like others who are asleep, but let us be alert and self-controlled. For those who sleep, sleep at night, and those who get drunk get drunk at night. . . ."

(I Thessalonians 5:6-8)

"Do not get drunk on wine, which leads to debauchery. Instead be filled with the Spirit."

(Ephesians 5:18)

"Therefore prepare your minds for action; be self-controlled. . . ."

(I Peter 1:13)

"Be self-controlled and alert."

(I Peter 5:8)

Contentions

"Do everything without arguing or complaining. . . ."

(Philippians 2:14)

Poor Priorities

"Seek first his Kingdom and his righteousness and all these things will be yours as well."

(Matthew 6:33)

Worry

"Do not worry about tomorrow, for tomorrow will worry about itself. Each day has enough trouble of its own."

(Matthew 6:34)

Anxiety

"Cast all your anxiety on him because He cares for you."

(I Peter 5:7)

"Do not be anxious about anything, but in everything, by prayer and petition, with thanksgiving, present your requests to God."

(Philippians 4:6)

Careless Use of Time

"Look carefully, then how you walk, not as unwise men, but as wise, making the most of the time, because the days are evil." (RSV)

(Ephesians 5:15)

Impatience

"We urge you, brothers, warn those who are idle, encourage the timid, help the weak be patient with everyone."

(I Thessalonians 5:14)

Basic Christian Life

The following verses are intended to aid a young Christian's growth so that "ye walk worthy of God who hath called you unto His kingdom and glory" (I Thessalonians 2:12) (KJV).

1. *The Bible*: (a) is the guide (Psalm 119:105), (b) to be studied (II Timothy 2:15), (c) to mediate on (Joshua 1:8–9), (d) to memorize (Psalm 119:9-11).
2. *Prayer*: (a) in God, the Father's name (John 14:13-14), (b) in order to receive (Matthew 21:22), (c) pray rather than worry (Philippians 4:6-7), (d) continually (Luke 18:1, I Thessalonians 5:17).
3. *Fellowship*: (a) because of being born again (I John 1:13), (b) to encourage one another (Hebrews 10:25), (c) continually (Acts 2:42).
4. *Witness*: (a) to all everywhere (Acts 1:8), (b) it is commanded (Matthew 28:19-20), (c) it is committed to each Christian (II Corinthians 5:19-20).
5. *Obedience*: (a) for God's sake (Romans 1:5), (b) obey above all else (I Samuel 15:22), (c) God has commanded it and it is best for each (Jeremiah 7:23).
6. *Holy Spirit*: (a) He comforts and teaches the Christian (John 14:26), (b) He dwells in Christians (I Corinthians 3:16), (c) Walk in Him (Galatians 5:16–17).

7. *Assurance*: The only way we know the type of a tree is by the fruit it bears. We are assured a tree is an apple tree because it has apples on it. The only way a Christian may be assured daily of their salvation is by their actions and fruit. The verses below are fruits of a saved man. "These things have I written unto you that believe on the name of the Son of God, that you may know that ye have eternal life" (I John 5:13) (KJV). Note: All references are from I John (KJV).

  (a) having fellowship with God and other believers (1:3, 7).
  (b) having joy (1:4).
  (c) confessing sin (1:9).
  (d) keeping His commandments (2:3, 3:23-24, 5:3).
  (e) keeping His word (2:5).
  (f) walking as Christ walked (2:6).
  (g) loving the brethren (2:10, 3:14, 23, 4:7, 12, 21).
  (h) remaining with believers (2:19).
  (i) practicing righteousness (2:29, 2:7, 9).
  (j) purifying self (3:3).
  (k) laying down our lives for the brethren (self-denial) (3:16).
  (l) loving in deed (3:18-19).
  (m) listening to believers (4:6).
  (n) abiding in love (4:16).

8. *Temptations*: (a) all temptations can be overcome (I Corinthians 10:13), (b) it builds you up (James 1:2-4), (c) those who overcome are rewarded (James 1:12).

9. *Promises of God's presence*: (a) be strong and courageous (Joshua 1:9), (b) it builds you up (James 1:2-4), (c) no one can harm you (Hebrews 13:5-6), to all who receive him (John 1:12).

10. *Promises of God's strength*: (a) to those who wait for Him (Psalms 27:14), (b) to those who need it (Isaiah 40:29-31), (c) to those who go to Him (Hebrews 4:16).

11. *Promises of God's victory*: (a) you can do all things (Philippians 4:13), (b) you can gain it through Jesus, His Son (I Corinthians 15:57-58), (c) it comes by faith (I John 5:4), (d) more than conquerors (Romans 8:37).

As a new Christian, you should also be very careful of the company you keep. "He that walketh with wise men shall be wise" (Proverbs 13:20); also, "his delight is in the law of the Lord/the Bible/and in His law doth he meditate day and night. And he shall be like a *tree* planted by the rivers of water, that bringeth forth his *fruit* in his season: his leaves also shall *not wither*, and whatsoever he doeth shall prosper" (Psalms 1:2-3). You are like the company you keep. Fellowship with the right company, and God will be pleased. In addition to this, remember that you will prosper and bear fruit only as you study and meditate on the Word of God.

Clarity of Clergy Concerns

Many of the clergy have not understood the personal responsibility and the disease concept aspect of treatment programs and of AA. I know of no program that teaches that the person is an innocent victim with no choice in what has become of their life. Rather, all programs stress individual recovery is a matter of personal responsibility and choice. By virtue of entering AA, the individual admits to their powerlessness over alcohol.

Events occurring in the course of drinking: Moral bankruptcy can occur for the alcoholic before even they know what has happened.

Alcoholism is not an excuse but is a cause of family crisis, family violence, crime and numerous sins against people close to the alcoholic. That everything from incest and homosexuality to hitting a spouse occurs is not news to the clergy. However, the initial step is to get the individual sober, since nothing can be accomplished prior to sobriety. The clergy needs to support the family emotionally during family crisis. Those clergymen who are informed are vital to the sanity and survival of the spouse and children.

For the elderly, the clergy is usually a most trusted and revered individual. This powerful trust can be used to intervene and assist.

Motivation for Recovery: These individuals are dying a slow death that is destructive to their family, their church, their community and their relationship to God. Why a person enters treatment is secondary. The key is to get them there with a commitment to at least stay through detox. The staff will take it from there. A most exciting sight is a sick, dying alcoholic making it to treatment accompanied by the person's clergyman and a family member. The clergy's advance meeting of the staff will facilitate the smooth admission.

Shouldn't the Church Cure This? When someone is in cardiac arrest, the clergy wouldn't give much consideration to assuming full responsibility for the person's recovery. This recovery will be wrought by God and a team of experts giving specific, prompt attention; so it is with alcoholism. Few clergymen have the time or knowledge to assume twenty-eight days of specialized treatment for a sick alcoholic, plus their families. The special knowledge required for safe detox, education, therapy, and aftercare rests with the experts.

However, all programs of competence both welcome and encourage clergy participation and are appreciative of all clergy involvement. In fact, most will be seen as angels of mercy after awhile. That such caring exists has surprised many clergymen. The success of treatment and AA are well known. Please, meet the staffs of local treatment centers. Attend an AA meeting. Most programs welcome concerned professionals sitting in on lectures. Family nights are for all who care for the drinker. Certainly, more of the clergy need to be numbered there.

Is the Church Responsible for Alcoholism in the Congregation? This is a fear that the clergy has expressed on occasion. No, the church is not responsible, the individual is. The church is only responsible when the individual and the family are known to be suffering and nothing is done to assist. Read Luke 10:25–37, which is commonly referred to as the Parable of the Good Samaritan. The first person to pass the man who was beaten was a priest who passed by on the other side (v.31). Too many men and women of God have passed the alcoholic by on the other side. Since alcoholism is all pervasive, most congregations have both alcoholics and the family of alcoholics. Each will require help to recover.

Certainly life has greater pleasures than picking up a down and out, smelly and sick alcoholic. Consider Matthew 25:31–46. The alcoholic certainly qualifies as the least of our brothers and sisters.

The challenge when disgusted and discouraged is to remember the worth of any one individual in God's eyes. Consider the passage "are not two sparrows sold for a penny? Yet not one of them will fall to the ground without the Father's will. But even the hairs of your head are all numbered. Fear not, therefore; you are of more value than many sparrows" (Matthew 10:29–31). Also, the parable in Luke of the angels who rejoice for the one lamb who is saved. We are commanded by God to serve the least of man. "Do not neglect to show hospitality to strangers, for thereby some have entertained angels unawares" (Hebrews 13:2).

What if We Doctrinally Disagree with a Point in the AA Philosophy or Treatment Program Philosophy? The debates between all three groups will never be fully settled. However, a respectful debate of issues is usually stimulating and useful. Since the positives of treatment far outweigh the uselessness of a drinking alcoholic, the clergy needs to examine exactly what the objections are. The AA program is a spiritual program. The steps state "God as we understand him." If the clergy is involved and loving, they can share much about God.

What if the Alcoholic Relapses? The issue here may well be one of forgiveness. Man is not exempt from doing what is worst for him. Thus, relapses will occur in about 30 percent of all persons who begin drinking again. This is disappointing and often hurts those who love the alcoholic. However, forgiveness is the key. The clergy must set the example of being quick to forgive and restore the person once they are again sober.

My hope and prayer is that these thoughts and Scriptures will inspire compassion, equip each to help facilitate recovery, and bring about cooperation for aiding those who suffer alcohol-related difficulties.

Chapter 14

ORGANIC BRAIN SYNDROMES

Kinds of OBS

DOUBTLESS, this general diagnosis is one that is frequently entered on patient's clinical, medical and legal records of elderly patients. Until recently, many state laws have enabled a family to place a patient with "organic brain syndrome" in a nursing home and then assume all legal and financial matters for the patient, needed or not.

The tragedy of this general diagnosis being so widely accepted is severalfold. First, OBS does not indicate what is wrong with the patient. Secondly, OBS is generally accepted as being irreversible, thus robbing the patient of *any* therapy. Thirdly, various types of OBS are in fact treatable. Even though the person cannot be cured, the person can often be restored to a functional level. Fourthly, OBS often carries with it a moral indictment. Statements by professional people and community people often indicate this patient "deserved" or "brought it on themselves," particularly if the individual has been previously diagnosed as an alcoholic.

The problem with this diagnosis is that a learned clinician does not know what is wrong with the client based on OBS being on the record. This diagnosis is often a cover for the physician's or psychiatrist's inability to know what is wrong with the patient and *THEIR APATHY IN FINDING OUT.* Diagnosis is by the very essence of all it entails suggests the treatment and the course of therapy. The diagnosis of OBS does not state:

1. What is the behavior seen?
2. What is the symptomotology?
3. What is the patient's level of functioning?
4. Based on the above, what does the doctor expect the support staff to do?
5. Etiology of the difficulty?
6. Duration of the difficulty?

These are vital points in the planning of treatment approaches and in the need of placement, if appropriate. Another point is that accurate diagnosis is obligatory for those medical and psychiatric personnel who assume this responsibility. A diagnosis of OBS which keeps an individual from receiving adequate treatment constitutes a violation of ethical and professional standards (and hence a charge of malpractice).

Some of the many types of OBS are listed below:

DISEASE	ETIOLOGY
Wernicke's encephalopathy	Alcoholism
Korsakoff's psychosis	Alcoholism
Alzheimer's disease	Unknown
Depression/grief	Significant loss/Poly drug usage
Cerebral vascular accident	Diabetes mellitus, Alcoholism
Intoxication	Alcoholism
Pre-senile dementia	Unknown
Parkinson's disease	Unknown
Pick's syndrome	
Marchiafava's disease	Alcoholism
Subdural hematoma	Fall, stroke
Carcinoma	Unknown; possible alcoholism
Nutritional deficiency	Alcoholism, lack of financial resources, Laxative usage

Alcohol–Related OBS and Behavior

Such a formidable list of OBS-type illnesses serves to reiterate the need for accurate diagnosis. Perhaps to further make this point, a discussion of each of these diseases is in order. Incidentally, eight* of the twelve disorders listed can be, and frequently are, a result of alcohol use or abuse.

WERNICKE'S ENCEPHALOPATHY*

Symptoms:
- Ataxia.
- Ocular abnormalities.
- Mental confusion.
- Profound disorientation.
- Often preceeds Korsakoff's syndrome.

Behaviors:
- Wandering.
- Forgetfulness.
- Does not improve dramatically when sober.
- Frequently gets lost.

KORSAKOFF'S PSYCHOSIS*

Symptoms:
- Memory impairment.
- Confabulation.
- Disorientation.
- Improvement is slow and limited.

Behaviors:
- Frequently unable to live alone/institution.
- Remote/Recent memory is impaired—can't remember vital information.

ALZHEIMER'S DISEASE

Described in four phases:

Phase I:
- Insidious loss of initiative.
- Angry outbursts.
- Stays only in familiar surroundings.
- Loss of interest in longstanding activities.
- Refuses to go out in public.
- Frequent display of temper.

Phase II:
- Slow speech and understanding.
- Unable to make decisions.
- Able to function in all ADL activities.
- Unable to complete specialized tasks, especially including arithmetic and logic.
- Starts a story and doesn't finish.
- Becomes introspective.
- Avoids many situations that used to be participated in and enjoyed.

Phase III:
- Obvious mental disability.
- Unable to complete ADL activities.
- Recent memory is failing.
- Remote memory is completely clear.
- Disoriented in familiar places.
- Unable to act appropriately in any setting.
- No orientation to time and place.
- Misidentifies known people.
- Unable to follow simple directions.

Phase IV:
- Unable to complete any ADL activity without assistance.
- Does not recognize any persons.
- Apathetic.

Recent memory is failing.
Remote memory is failing.

Unable to be alone without
becoming lost.
Unable to state who they are.

DEPRESSION*

Loss of interest in activities.
Sleep disturbance.
Appetite disturbance.
Unable to concentrate.
Inability to complete simple
or routine tasks.
Somatic concerns.

Restless.
Becomes readily angry or anxious.
Rapid weight loss/gain.
Lethargic.

CEREBRAL VASCULAR ACCIDENT*

Aphasia.
Loss of balance.
Loss of concentration.
Headaches.
Loss of consciousness.
Possible paralysis.
Stuperous.

Unable to say many words.
Complains of pain.
Despair and fear.
Slow to react.
Seeks only the familiar.

ACUTE INTOXICATION/WITHDRAWAL*

Loss of consciousness.
Stuperous.
Possible paralysis.
Loss of balance.
Tremors.

High BAC (150/100 or higher).
Unable to speak plainly.
Slow to react.

PRE-SENILE DEMENTIA*

Confusion.
Poor recent memory.
Not related to physical
difficulties.
Person is under age sixty.

Seeks only the familiar.

PARKINSON'S DISEASE

Tremors.

Dependence on medications for
relief.

MARCHIAFAVA'S DISEASE

Degeneration of the corpus
callosum.
Mental malfunction (memory
loss).
Diagnosable mostly at autopsy.

Wandering.
Loss of orientation to time, place,
person.

CARCINOMA*

Headaches.	Pain relief sought.
Light flashes behind eyes.	Confused conversation of a
Confusion.	transitory nature.
Disorientation.	Irritable.

NUTRITIONAL DEFICIENCY*

Dehydration.	Beri-Beri.
Poor eyesight.	Hunger.
Baggy clothes.	Stealing of food.

Domiciliary Care

For the victims of Korsakoff's and Wernicke's syndromes, the habilitation concept has been ably and successfully demonstrated. Unlike the Alzheimer's victim, which requires total care in the stages of their illness, Korsakoff–Wernicke victims are not as debilitated. The debilitating aspect of this illness is seen in symp-. toms such as recent memory impairment. For example, the person may not remember breakfast or taking their medication. But this person can shower, clean up, dress, feed self and the commonly accepted activities of daily living. The domiciliary care program provides assistance to the brain-affected alcoholic. This program is providing humanistic caring to these people while removing them from the streets.

Chapter 15

CAUSES OF EXCESS MORTALITY DUE TO ALCOHOL USE/ALCOHOLISM

Statistical Data

PROFESSIONALS in the field of alcoholism have long contended that the untreated disease will result in death or insanity. This chapter demonstrates the major causes of excess mortality due to alcoholism; that is, natural death, accidental alcohol deaths, homocide and suicide.

Because so many alcoholics are recovering, enough special attention has not been given to the issue of alcoholic sudden death. Many factors influence who will die from alcohol abuse. Included factors are: more unmarried persons die alcohol-related deaths than those who are married; urban alcoholics die more frequently than rural alcoholics; middle socioeconomic class alcoholics die more frequently than either the lower or higher socioeconomic classes (Mellor, 1975). Natural alcohol-related deaths are also influenced by many factors: genetic trends, stress occupation, ethnic group and family size (Mellor, 1975; Day, 1976).

These various factors are those from which excess mortality data are drawn. When discussing excess mortality, the number-one cause of death is alcoholism, including both natural death and accidental death. Excess mortality are those who die in addition to the general population mortality; in other words, premature death. The alcohol excess mortality rate is estimated to be 28 persons per every 1,000 of the population (HEW, 1975). Other estimates of excess mortality, if the classification for heavy drinkers is 3 drinks consumed two or more times weekly for the males between 30–70 years of age, then the mortality rate is 12 deaths/1,000. If consumption is 4 drinks two or more times a week, then the excess mortality rate is 79/1,000. In the study reporting 12/1,000, 83 percent of the premature deaths were by 15 years or more, while 48.3 percent among the 79/1,000 deaths were 15 years earlier then if alcohol had not been involved (Day, 1976). Also, important to note, in deaths in which secondary cause is alcohol consumption (i.e. suicide, homicide and accidents), these rates rise dramatically (Day, 1976).

When discussing the excess mortality of women, one study reports women die approximately half the rate of men (Dahlgren and Mayrhed, 1977). Causes of death included violence, suicide and respiratory disease in equal numbers and cirrhosis of the liver approximately three times as great (Dahlgren and Mayrhed, 1977).

Major Categories of Excess Mortality Deaths due to Alcohol

Natural Deaths. Finkle (1976) documents a study of 53 million deaths in 18 United States cities; of these, 1,022 propoxyphene-related deaths (Darvon primarily) were identified. These deaths were prescription drug and/or alcohol caused. Forty-six percent were suicides and 26 percent were classified as accidental deaths. The most commonly encountered drug besides alcohol was diazepam (29% of all cases).

Edward's study documents deaths due to tuberculosis, cancer (breast, pharynx, lung, digestive tract), various heart conditions, cerebral bleeding and embolism, arteriosclerosis, pneumonia, cirrhosis, and accidents. By far, accidents and heart disease were the two major causes of alcoholic deaths.

In Perper's discussion of sudden death, two major concerns are stated. One is that many of these people were in hospital emergency rooms and, because of their intoxicated state and absence of apparent trauma, they were released without treatment. Many head injuries are attributed to the patient's intoxication. Many others will die in jail cells of subdural hematomas or internal hemorrhage (either spleen or liver). He also discusses those who died of methanol poisoning when using these substances to prevent withdrawal.

Fire Deaths. Systematic study is rarely done on this category of death. Of the 12,000 who die annually, approximately four-fifths are alcohol impaired at the time of death. Alcohol, then, is the underlying cause of death, although it may not be the primary cause of the fatal fire. The probability of death increases with the consumption of alcohol, beginning at a 0.05 blood alcohol level. The consumption of alcohol coupled with smoking is the greatest single cause of fire (Hollis, 1974). Another study reports that men are impaired twice as often as women, are likely under fifty, and the time of the fire is usually a weekend night.

Motorcycle Deaths. One study seemed representative of the findings: of ninety-nine fatalities, sixty-two autopsies included the victim's BAL, two-thirds (41) had measurable BALs, and one-half (32) had illegally high BALs at the time of death. (0.10 or higher). Almost all drivers were 20–34 years old (Baker and Fisher, 1977).

Aviation Accidents. The FAA reports of general aviation accidents show that in 1977, 16 percent of the 21,966 accidents were fatal (or 3,433 crashes resulted in fatalities). Of those pilots, 81 percent had BALs of greater than 0.10 at the time of death (Lacefield et al. 1978). Another study reports that the altitude increases that a pilot undergoes can raise the BAL without the pilot ingesting any more alcohol. While the data was not conclusive, it does raise areas for further investigation (Higgins et al. 1970).

Motor Vehicle Deaths. This category is by far the most documented and best supported by statistics and research. Several studies link driver's BALs to evidence of arteriosclerotic heart disease at the time of fatal accident. Significantly, all white drivers in the age 49–60 age class had artery damage and/or evidence of an infarction (Baker and Spitz, 1970) at the time they caused the accident. Of those not at fault, the same percentage had heart disease, but only 13 percent had any measurable BALs.

In Waller's study, he discovered that the age-related drinking factor was strikingly different. Of the crashes of the group under

20 years of age, half had been drinking and half had not. Significantly, in the 20–40 age class, almost every driver had been drinking and the crashes occurred almost exclusively in the nighttime hours. Most drivers in the 25–59 age class had been drinking, and approximately one of every four crashed in the daytime. The persons aged 60 or older almost never had been drinking and tended to crash during the day. Approximately 28 percent of these drivers studied were considered by physiological condition at autopsy (no arrest record, etc.) to be social drinkers, while 47 percent were presumed to be problem drinkers.

Haberman and Baden report in their study that one-fourth of all motor vehicle fatalities are known alcoholics. Of that number, 38 percent are drivers, 16 percent are passengers, and 21 percent are pedestrians.

The National Safety Council statistics indicate that 250,000 people have died in the last decade on American highways. Additionally, 6.5 million families have had at least one member of their families injured seriously during the same time period.

Other Accidental Deaths. Schmidt and deLint reported on 85 excess mortality deaths in their San Francisco study. In every category, the expected deaths far exceeded the actual deaths. These categories include railway and water transport 0 to 6, ex-3; accidental poisoning 0 to 20, ex-1.3; accidental falls 0 to 18, ex-31; accidents caused by fire 0 to 31, ex-1.3; homicide 0 to 3, ex-7; other accidents 0 to 8, ex-6.5; motor vehicle traffic 0 to 17, ex-11.7. The excess mortality from these accidents are attributable to the alcohol ingested, life-style and conditions of the alcoholic, as well as their personality characteristics.

Haberman and Baden also report on motor vehicle accidents. Of those dying in falls, 41 percent had a BAL of 0.10 or higher, 46.4 percent of fire deaths and 53 percent of all drowning victims had a BAL of 0.10 or above.

Homicides. Homicides occur daily throughout the country. Tremendous amounts of time and money are spent prosecuting those who are guilty of homicide. However, the story invariably includes alcohol use/abuse.

Day (1977) reports that of the 21,310 homicides reported in 1975 probably as high as 70 percent were related to alcohol or

14,917. The state of Florida and NIAAA statistics indicate that the figure may be as high as 90 percent.

While alcohol influence is not an excuse to escape prosecution, the involvement of alcohol in these deaths must be reported with greater consistency.

Suicides. Suicide is becoming one of the major problems of the elderly. While younger persons average one successful suicide for every seven attempts, in persons over sixty-five years old the ratio becomes one successful suicide for every two attempts (active suicides). For passive suicide, no accurate information can ever be fully attained. Passive suicides are deaths that result when someone quits eating or refuses to follow through on life-sustaining medication regimens.

While younger persons are concerned with using a suicidal gesture to impact on someone else, often the older person has no significant person to impress. Several researchers have verified that when suicide is not directed at affecting someone, the attempt is much more likely to be successful (Dorpat and Boswell, 1963).

Alcohol usage dulls reason and judgment and makes problems appear much larger/bleaker than at other times. Thus, suicides, particularly successful attempts, most frequently occur under alcohol's influence. Some indication of how ethanol can enhance an attempt are those by violent means. As homicides under such circumstances are considered "crimes of passion," no such attitude exists for suicide cases.

Methods of committing suicide are the same for all age groups. A method receiving more interest at the present is the single car against a pole or tree "accident." This method of suicide places an acceptable cause of death on the death certificate and removes the stigma of a suicide for family and friends. Other methods for men are guns, knives, jumping off cliffs and buildings, and means which show little concern for the condition of the body after death. Women tend to be much more concerned and prefer gas, pills and such means. Any of these means insure lethality when combined with ethanol.

Other Information and Case Histories

As one author stated, "The characteristics of alcoholics—their

drinking behavior, smoking habits, emotional state and life-style—
are uniquely expressed in their mode of dying" (Revzin, 1978).

Whichever mode of dying is discussed, the alcoholic's drinking
is either evident (as in cirrhosis) or indicated (as in fires). The
statistics presented in this section only touch on the issues of
deaths of problem drinkers, significant others and innocent other
persons who die as a result of the alcohol consumption of another.
Until better systems of reporting these deaths are required by law,
statistics will never adequately reflect the number of persons
dying from alcohol-related causes in the United States yearly.

Treatment and prevention funding is proportionate to the
magnitude of a given problem, and the social and political pressure applied for action against that problem. When the magnitude
of excess alcohol mortality is fully understood, funding must
result to deal with all facets of this crucial problem.

Following are actual histories taken (or combined) from news-
paper accounts of those who die alcohol deaths. They are most
representative of the reasons and circumstances under which
people die.

People Who Die Alcohol-Related Deaths

Mr. J had been sober for well over two years. After becoming
close to a "skid row" alcoholic following his retirement, this
distinguished gentleman had provided leadership to many
struggling to achieve sobriety. Mr. J was staunchly religious
and active in both AA and the local church. He befriended
many of the men no one else would befriend. He was 68 when
he died in his sleep of a heart attack.

Mrs. L was a well-known individual. Unlike Mr. J, she was not
an alcoholic; in fact, her career rarely permitted indulgence in
drinking. She was happily married and had three lovely daughters. Following a celebration, she "inexplicably" drowned in
a rather freakish accident. However, it was an accident she
could not deal with because she had been drinking earlier in
the evening.

Most drownings can be traced directly to alcohol consump-
tions. More commonly, the death is a fisherman who's imbibed
while waiting for a "catch."

Mrs. P was a young, attractive divorcee with three children. She was a crackerjack legal secretary and was proud to support her children. Going home from work, her car was hit from behind by an intoxicated driver of a pickup truck. As she started to leave her car, the same driver trying to leave the scene of the accident ran her over and killed her.

As is often the case in an alcohol-related death, the individual(s) killed were not the ones drinking. They are just as dead. People like this die frequently because:

1. Legislation is not tough enough to make the penalty fit the circumstance.
2. People who drink foolishly and erroneously believe they are capable of driving.
3. Before any driver can be licensed they should be required to watch a film on drinking and driving consequences. Once a driver reaches remedial driver's training, it could well be too late for an innocent person.

Mr. I had been a " skid row" alcoholic for numerous years. He frequently dried out and made a serious commitment to sobriety, only to begin drinking again within weeks. One afternoon he came by the treatment center office and requested to go into town. As was often the case, he did not return that evening. A few days later he was found propped up in the alley behind the lounge he frequented, with a partial drink in his hand, dead!

Mr. W was in the treatment program for almost a year. During that time he was sober a great deal of the time, although if one of the other guys began drinking around the grounds, he would drink with them. He always went peaceably to bed and was never really a cause of problems. In fact, the only time he was not quiet was when his disability checks were due. He began receiving them while at the center but had become increasingly sensitive about paying his way before receiving the balance. This led to his decision to leave the treatment program. Predictably, he began to drink shortly thereafter. As he decompensated back into uncontrolled drinking, his check began to support only drinking. Police allege he shot the landlord to death while drinking because he believed the landlord had stolen his money.

Mr. W faces second-degree murder charges. People rarely commit murder while sober.

Mr. Q was a devoted family man. He loved his son and many were the Sundays the two spent watching pro football games and drinking beer. One Sunday Mr. Q made a remark that the halfback was not worth the money the team was paying. The son took exception to the statement and an argument began. The argument ended when the elder Mr. Q, then 56, shot to death the son, who was 23. Had either been sober (later, police would determine both men had BALs above 0.10), the senseless tragedy would easily have been prevented.

Mr. B was an elderly gentleman with a distinguished and respected career. He was now alone but employed a housekeeper. Not known as a heavy drinker, on this evening he had been drinking throughout the time. As best the police can piece together, Mr. B had begun to dress for bed when he somehow lost his balance and fell, striking his head on a night table. The combination of the blow to his head and a BAL estimated at 0.15 caused Mr. B's death.

Mrs. K had been widowed for some six years as her seventy-second birthday was celebrated. Although slight in build, she figured two drinks at her birthday party would be harmless (combined with her arthritis medication produced synergism and a high degree of intoxication). Her family took her home, saw to it she was safely in bed and left. Police say the fire started in a frayed electrical cord on a kitchen appliance. Mrs. K burned to death—she was unable to comprehend the situation and escape the fire—and was found in what remained of her bed.

Mr. O had become increasingly despondent after retirement and the death of his wife of forty-two years. Despite his children's support and concern, and treatment for depression at a local mental health center, Mr. O decided life was not worth living! He had never taken a drink with an aspirin, but tonight he drank most of a six pack of beer and then swallowed his bottle of anti-depressant medications. He was found dead two days later.

Mrs. A fell and broke her hip on an ice-slick sidewalk outside her apartment building. Despite the efforts of her two daughters, she was placed in a nursing home to recover. Eighty-one-year-old women heal most slowly from so serious an accident. As the hip healed, the severe pain subsided and Mrs. A began walking with a walker. If she was up too long on her hip, the pain was bad but bearable. She was discharged from the nursing home with a Darvon prescription. Her daughters threw a huge celebration and invited long-time family friends. To make sure she'd feel good, she took one Darvon capsule. During the party she had two small champagne glasses of "that delightful bubbly." One hour later she was dead, the victim of an accidental overdose. Darvon and ethyl alcohol are responsible for many accidental overdoses.

These ten cases were people like every other. The causes of death were premature and tragic. Only three of the persons who died were alcoholics. The others died under the cruelty of alcohol combined with carelessness, ignorance and circumstance. These seven people and all those like them die from a highly preventable cause of death.

Concluding Information and Data

As stated, but recapped in closing, are the statistics provided by the National Council on Alcoholism, NIAAA, and the state of Florida. Remember, these are alcohol-related, not limited to alcoholics.

Fire deaths	80%	
Drownings	70%	
Home accidents	32%	
Falls	77%	
Motor Vehicle Deaths	59% (at least 30,000 people)	
Pedestrian Accidents	36%	
Suicides by Alcoholics	33%	
Suicides by non-alcoholics	85%	(combined 35,000 people)
Homicides by alcoholics	25–30%	

Homicides by non-
  alcoholics   85–90%
Cirrhosis of liver   95% are alcoholics (approx. 30,000)

The above statistics only refer to deaths, not those having serious injury. Perhaps visualizing 35,000 people is surrealistic. This means that every 14 minutes of every day, someone impaired by alcohol successfully commits suicide. Every 17 minutes someone impaired by alcohol is involved in a fatal accident. This is every hour of every day throughout the year!

Inordinate numbers of studies are done every year on what might cause cancer and what should be avoided. Yet, alcohol abuse is killing this number of Americans, and the alcohol/alcoholism research and treatment funds are often the first in budget cuts.

How many must die before a lasting solution is found?

BIBLIOGRAPHY

Adams, J.E.: *The Christian Counselor's Manual*. New Jersey Presbyterian and Reformed Publishing Co., Nutley City, N.J., 1973.

Alcohol Education and Training News. "Alcohol Abuse and the Older Person." Department of Health and Rehabilitative Services, Florida, 1978.

"Alcohol Problems Among the Elderly." *Bottom Line*, Spring, 1978, 4-9.

Amaducci, L., et al. (Eds.): *Aging of the Brain and Dementia*. New York: Raven Press, 1980.

Anderson, D.J.: *Anxiety/Conflicts and Chemical Dependency*. Minneapolis: Hazelden Foundation, 1976.

Anonymous. My psychiatrist, AA, and me. *AA Grapevine, 22(3):*38-39, 1965.

Alcoholics Anonymous. "This is A.A." New York General Service Office, 1953.

Armor, D.J.; Johnson, P.; Polich, S.; and Stambul, H.: "Trends in U.S. Adult Drinking Practices." Summary report prepared for National Institute on Alcohol Abuse and Alcoholism under Contract No. ADM 281-76-0020. Santa Monica: Rand Corporation. February, 1977.

Bacon, S.D.: Traffic accidents involving alcoholism in the USA: Second-stage aspects of a social problem. *Q J Studies Alcohol, 39:*1133; 1979.

Baker, S.P., and Fisher, R.S.: Alcohol and motorcycle fatalities. *Am J Public Health, 67:*246-249, 1977.

Baker, S.P., and Spitz, W.U.: Age and blood counts in fatal accident drivers. *JAMA, 214*(6):1079-1088, 1977.

Barnes, B.F., et al.: Problems of families caring for Alzheimer's patients. Use of a support group. *J Am Geriatr Soc, 29:*80-85, 1981.

Barns, Eleanor, Sack, Ann, and Shore, Herbert: Guidelines to treatment approaches: Modalities and methods for use with the aged. *Gerontologist, 13:*513-527, 1973.

Bartol, Mari Anne: Nonverbal communications in patients with Alzheimer's disease. *J Gerontol Nurs, 5:*21-31, 1979.

Bell, P., and Evans, J.: *Counseling the Black Client: Alcohol Use and Abuse in Black America*. Center City, Minnesota Hazelden Foundation, 1981.

213

Bergman, K., Foster, E.M., and Matthews, V.: Management of the demented elderly patient in the community. *Br J Psychiatry, 132*:441–449, 1978.

Billings, E.E., Wick, R.L., Gerle, R.J., and Chase, R.C.: Effects of alcohol on pilot performance during instrument flight. *FAA, AM-72-4:* 5-67, 1972.

Blum, E.M., and Blum, R.H.: *Alcoholism: Modern Psychological Approaches to Treatment.* San Francisco: Jossey–Bass, 1976.

Blumberg, L., Shipley, T.E., Shandler, I.W.: *Skid Row and Its Alternatives.* Philadelphia: Temple University Press, 1973.

Brink, T.L.: The battle against senility. *Mental Hygiene, 61*:10–11, 1977.

Brody, J.A., and Mills, G.S.: On considering alcohol as a risk factor in specific diseases. *Am J Epidemiology, 107*:462–466, 1978.

Brunn, K., et al.: *Alcohol Control Policies in Public Health Perspective.* New Jersey: Rutgers Center of Alcohol Studies, 1975, p. 942.

Burnside, I.M.: *Nursing and the Aged.* New York: McGraw–Hill, 1976.

Burnside, Irene Mortenson: Alzheimer's disease: An overview. *J Gerontol Nurs, 5*:14–20, 1979.

Butt, W.R.: *Hormone Chemistry,* 2nd ed. New York: John Wiley and Sons, 1975, vol. I.

Carruth, Bruce, et al.: *Lifestyles, Drinking Practices and Drinking Problems of Older Alcoholics.* New Brunswick, New Jersey: Rutgers Center of Alcohol Studies, 1973.

Casper, R., and Mozerskey: Social correlates of drinking and driving. *Quad J Stud Alc, 39*:85–99, 1978.

Chantan, F.B.: Therapeutic supports for the patient with OBS. *Geriatrics, 35*:100–102, 1980.

Charatan, F.B.: Acute confusion and the elderly. *Hospital Physician,* May, 1976.

Choosing a Nursing Home for the Person with Intellectual Loss. Burke Rehabilitation Center, White Plains, New York, p. 4.

Cook, R.H.: Memory loss in Alzheimer's disease. *Annals of Neurology, 5*: 105–106, 1979.

Corkin, Suzanne, et al. (Eds.): *Alzheimer's Disease: A Report of Progress in Research.* New York: Raven Press, 1981.

Curlee, J.: Alcoholism and the empty nest. *Bulletin of the Menninger Clinic, 33*:165–71, 1969.

Dahlgren, L., and Myrhed, M.R.: Alcoholic females II: Causes of death with reference to sex difference. *Acta Psychiat Scand, 56*:81–91, 1977.

Day, N.: Estimates of the role of alcoholism mortality. *Drinking and Drug Practice Surveyor* (reprint).

DeBoni, U., and McLacklan, D.R.C., et al.: Senile dementia and Alzheimer's disease: A current view. *Life Science, 27*:1–14, 1980.

Dobbie, J.: Substance abuse among the elderly. *Addictions,* (Fall):5, 1977.

Do It Now Foundation: *What Senior Citizens Should Know About Alcohol and Drugs.* Phoenix, Ar., 1978.

Dorpat, T.L., and Boswell, J.W.: An evaluation of suicidal intent and suicidal attempts. *Comprehensive Psychiatry, 4*:114-125, 1963.

Drew, Leslie: Alcoholism as a self-limiting disease. *Quarterly Journal of Studies on Alcohol*, (December):956-967, 1968.

Drews, T.R.: *Getting Them Sober*. New Jersey: Haven Books, 1980.

Edwards. G., Kule. E., Nichols, P., Taylor, C.: Alcoholism and correlates of mortality: Implications for epidemiology. *J of Studies on Alcohol, 39* (9):1607-1617, 1978.

Clark, M., Hager. M., and Shapiro, D.: Epidemic of Senility: Alzheimer's Disease or Presenile Dementia. *Newsweek, 5,* November 1979, p. 95.

Faberlow, N.L.: *The Many Faces of Suicide: The Accident Process*. New York: McGraw-Hill, 1980.

Finkle, B.S., et al.: A national assessment of propoxyphene in postmortem medicolegal investigation, 1972-1975. *J Forens Sci, 21*:706-742, 1976.

Florida Department of Health and Rehabilitative Services: *Shattering Myths about Drinking*. State of Florida, 1977.

Forrest, G.G.: *The Diagnosis and Treatment of Alcoholism*, 2nd ed. Springfield: Thomas, 1978.

Fox, R.: A multidisciplinary approach to the treatment of alcoholism. *American Journal of Psychiatry, 123*:769-778, 1967.

French L.A., and Hornbuckle, J.: Alcoholism among native Americans: An analysis. *Soc Work*, (July):275-280, 1980.

Fuller J. et al.: Dementia: Supportive groups for relatives. *British Medical Journal, 23*:1864-1885, 1979.

Funkhouser, M.J.: Identifying alcohol problems among elderly hospital patients. *Alcohol Health & Research World*, (Winter):28-34, 1977-78.

Getze, Linda: They're coping with senility. *Modern Maturity*, (April):82-85, 1981.

Glasscote, R.M., et al.: The treatment of alcoholism: A study of programs and problems. Washington: American Psychiatric Association, 1967.

Gust. D.: *Up, Down, and Sideways on Wet and Dry Booze*. Minneapolis: CompCare Publications, 1977.

Guttman D.: *A Study of Legal Drug Use by Older Americans*. U.S. Government Printing Office, 1977.

Haberman, P.W., and Baden, M.M.: *Alcohol, Other Drugs and Violent Death*. New York: Oxford University, Press, 1978.

Harford T.C.: The Distribution of Alcohol Consumption in Metropolitan Boston by day of week. Unpublished manuscript, 1977.

Harvard Medical School Health Letter. "Moderation versus Abuse or How Much Alcohol is Safe?" Volume 8 No. 2, 1981.

Hatsukami. D., and Pickens, R.: *Depression and Alcoholism*. Center City, Minnesota: Hazelden Foundation, 1980.

Hayman. M.: Current attitudes to alcoholism of psychiatrists in Southern California. *American Journal of Psychiatry, 112*:485-593, 1956.

Hayman, M.: *Alcoholism: Mechanism and Management*. Springfield: Thomas, 1966.

Hayter, Jean: Patients who have Alzheimer's disease. *American Journal of Nursing, 74*:1460–1463, 1974.

Hegarty, C.: *Alcoholism Today: The Progress and the Promise*. Minneapolis: CompCare Publications, 1979.

Hess, P., and Day, C.: *Understanding the Aging Patient*. Bowie, Maryland: Robert Brady Co., 1977.

Heston, L.L., et al.: "A Family Study of Alzheimer's Disease and Senile Dementia: An Interim Report." Proceedings of the Annual Meeting of the American Psychopathology Association, *69*:63–72, 1980.

Heston, Leonard, Mastri, Angelina, and Anderson, Eliring: Dementia of the Alzheimer type: Clinical genetics, natural history, and associated conditions. *Archives of General Psychiatry, 38*:1085–1090, 1981.

Higgins, E.A., Vaughan, J.A., and Funkhouser, G.E.: Blood Alcohol Concentrations as Affected by Combinations of Alcoholic Beverage Dosages and Altitudes (FAA-AM-70-5). Springfield, VA: Federal Aviation Administration, April, 1970, pp. 1–8.

Hoffman, F.G.: *Handbook on Drug and Alcohol Abuse. The Biomedical Aspects*. New York: Oxford University Press, 1975.

Hollis, W.S.: Fire deaths and drinking. *Alcohol Health and Research World*, NIAAA, (Summer):8–10, 1974.

Hurlock, Elizabeth B.: *Developmental Psychology*. New York: McGraw-Hill, 1968, p. 793ff.

Iskrant A.P., and Joliet, P.V.: *Accidents and Homicide*. Cambridge: Harvard University Press, 1968.

Johnson, V.E.: *I'll Quit Tomorrow*. New York: Harper and Row, 1973.

Kaplan, D.M., Smith, A., Grobstein, S.E., and Fischman, S.E.: Family mediation of stress. *Social Work, 18*:60–69, 1973.

Katz, Barbara: The struggle against senility. *Discover*, (November):62–64, 1980.

Katzman, Robert (Ed.): *Alzheimer's Disease: Senile Dementia and Related Disorders*. New York: Raven Press, 1977.

Keane, Evelyn E.: *Coping with Senility: A Guidebook*. Pittsburgh: COBS Publishing.

Kinney, J., and Leaton, Gwen: *Loosening the Grip: A Handbook of Alcohol Information*. St. Louis: C.V. Mosby, 1978.

Kissen, B., and Begleiter, H. (Eds.): *The Biology of Alcoholism: Clinical Pathology*. New York: Plenum, 1974, vol. 3.

Klein, R., Dean, A., and Bogdonoff, M.: The impact of illness upon the spouse. *Journal of Chronic Diseases, 20*:241–248, 1967.

Lacefield, D.J., Roberts, P.A., and Blossom, C.W.: Agricultural Aviation Versus Other General Aviation: Toxicological Findings in Fatal Accidents (FAA-AM-78-31). Oklahoma City, OK: Federal Aviation Administration, September 1978, pp. 1–5.

LaBarge, Emily: Counseling patients with senile dementia of the Alzheimer's type and their families. *The Personnel and Guidance Journal*, (November):139–142, 1981.

LaVorgna, D.: Group treatment for wives of patients with Alzheimer's disease. *Social Work in Health Care, 5*:219–221, 1979.

Lawton, M.P.: "Psychosocial and Environmental Approaches to the Care of Senile Dementia Patients." Proceedings of the Annual Meeting of the American Psychopathology Association, *69*:265–280, 1980.

Lazarus, L.W., et al.: A pilot study of an Alzheimer's patient's relatives discussion group. *Gerontologist, 39:*592–598, 1978.

Lezak. M.: Living with the characterologically altered brain impaired patient. *Journal of Clinical Psychiatry, 39*:592–598, 1978.

Luff, Marilyn: "The Agony of Alzheimer's." *Kiwanis Magazine,* August, 1981.

Mace. Nancy, and Rabins, P.V.: *The Thirty-Six Hour Day: A Family Guide to Caring for Persons with Memory Loss in Later Life, Alzheimer's Disease, and Other Dementing Illnesses.* Baltimore: Johns Hopkins Press, 1981.

"Managing the Person with Intellectual Loss (Demential or Alzheimer's Disease) at Home. Burke Rehabilitation Center, White Plains, New York.

"Management Guide on Alcoholism." Kemper Insurance Companies, Illinois, 1977.

"Manual on Alcoholism." American Medical Association, Illinois 1977.

Marden, Parker G.: "Alcohol Abuse and the Aged." Rockville, MD: National Institute on Alcohol Abuse and Alcoholism, 1976, p. 3.

Maxwell, R.: *The Booze Battle.* New York: Ballantine Books, 1976.

McCuster. C., Cherubin, C., and Zinberg, S.: Prevalence of alcoholism in a general municipal hospital population. *N.Y. State Mej, 71*:751–754, 1971.

Mellor, C.S.: The epidemiology of alcoholism. *Brit J of Psychiat, 9*:252–262. 1975.

Miller. Nancy E., and Cohen, Gene D. (Eds.): *Clinical Aspects of Alzheimer's Disease and Senile Dementia.* New York: Raven Press, 1981.

Mishara, B.L., and Kastenbaum, R.: *Alcohol and Old Age.* New York: Grune and Stratton. 1980.

Mishara, B.L., Kastenbaum, R., Baker, F., and Patterson, R.D.: Alcohol effects in old age: An experimental investigation. *Soc Sci Med, 9*(10): 535–547, 1975.

Mortimer. James; and Schuman, Leonard (Eds.): *The Epidemiology of Dementia.* New York: Oxford University Press, 1981.

Nandy, Kalidas (Ed.): *Senile Dementia: A Biomedical Approach.* New York: Elsevier/North Holland Biomedical Press, 1981.

National Clearinghouse on Alcohol Information. "National Death Rates." Rockville, MD: 1979. p 6.

Noble, E.P.: National Institute on Alcohol Abuse and Alcoholism: 3rd annual Report to Congress. June "Special Population Groups" 1978, pp. 17-25.

Ibid."Alcohol and Mortality." Jan. 1977.

Perper, J.A.: Sudden unexpected death in alcoholics. *Alcohol Health and Research World*, (Winter):18-26, 1974/75.

National Institute on Alcohol Abuse and Alcoholism: "Fact Sheet: Alcohol and the Elderly." Rockville Maryland, 1976, p. 4.

Neugarten, B.L.: Personality change in late life: A developmental perspective. In Eisdorfer, C., and Lawton, M.P. (Eds.): *The Psychology of Adult Development and Aging*. Washington: American Psychological Assoc., 1973.

Neugarten, B.L.: The future and the young–old. *Gerontologist, 15*(1, pt.2):4-9, 1975.

Neugarten, B.L.: Personality and aging. In Birren, J.E., and Schaie, K.W. (Eds.): *Handbook of the Psychology of Aging*. New York: Van Nostrand Reinhold, 1977.

Neugarten, B.L. et al.: *Personality in Middle and Late Life*. New York: Atherton, 1964.

Neugarten, B.L., and Gutmann, D.L.: Age-sex roles and personality in middle age: A thematic apperception study. In Neugarten, B.L. (Ed.): *Middle Age and Aging: A Reader in Social Psychology*. Chicago: University of Chicago Press, 1968.

Pfeiffer, E.: A short portable mental status questionnaire for the assessment of organic brain deficit in elderly patients. *Journal of the American Geriatrics Society, 23*:433-439, 1975a.

Pfeiffer, E.: *Functional Assessment: The OARS Multidimensional Functional Assessment Questionnaire*. Durham, N.C.: Duke University Center for the Study of Aging and Human Development, 1975b.

Pfeiffer, E.: Psychopathology and social pathology. In Birren, J.E., and Schaie, K.W. (Eds.): *Handbook of Psychology and Aging*. New York: Van Nostrand Reinhold, 1977.

Pfeiffer, E., Verwoerdt, A., and Wang, H.S.: Sexual behavior in aged men and women. I. Observations on 254 community volunteers. *Archives of General Psychiatry, 19*:753-758, 1968.

Pfeiffer, E., Verwoerdt, A., and Wang, H.S.: The natural history of sexual behavior in a biologically advantaged group of aged individuals. *Journal of Gerontology, 24*:193-198, 1969.

Pfeiffer, E., and Davis, G.C.: Determinants of sexual behavior in middle and old age. *Journal of the American Geriatrics Society, 20*:151-158, 1972.

Pfeiffer, E., and Busse, E.W.: Mental disorders in later life–affective disorders: Paranoid, neurotic and situational reactions. In Busse, E.W., and Pfeiffer, E. (Eds.): *Mental Illness in Later Life*. Washington: American Psychiatric Association, 1973.

Pawlak, V.J., Frazier, D.J., and Gray, N.: *Utilizing the Non-Disease Concept of Alcoholism in Community Education.* Phoenix: Do It Now Foundation, 1975.

Rathbone-McCuan, E., and Triegaardt, J.: The older alcoholic and the family. *Alcohol Health and Research World,* (Summer):7-12, 1979.

Reading, A.: "The Role of the General Hospital in a Community Alcoholism Program." Proc 3rd Ann Alcoholism Conf NIAAA, 1974, pp. 254-266.

Revzin, A.M.: "Effects of Ethanol on Visual Unit Activity in the Thalmus (FAA-AM-78-2). Oklahoma City, OK: Department of Transportation, January 1978, pp. 2-6.

Rosen, A., and Glatt, M.M.: Alcohol excess in the elderly. *QJ Stud Alcohol* 29:956-967, 1968.

Rosin, and Glatt: Alcohol excess in the elderly. *Quarterly Journal of Studies on Alcohol, 32*:53-59, 1971.

Ross, Jack: Alcoholics anonymous. *Journal of the Kansas Medical Society, 66*:23-27, 1965.

Saxon, S.V., and Etten, M.J.: *Physical Change and Aging.* New York: Tiresias Press, 1978.

Schuckit, M.A.: Geriatric alcoholism and drug abuse. *Gerontologist, 17*:168-174, 1977.

Schmidt, W., and deLint, J.: Causes of deaths in alcoholics. *Quart J Stud Alc, 33*:171-185, 1972.

Scott, E.M.: The technique of psychotherapy with alcoholics. *Quarterly Journal of Studies on Alcohol, 22*:69-80, 1961.

Shanas, E.: The family as social support systems in old age. *The Gerontologist, 19*:169-174, 1979.

Schuckit, M.A.: Geriatric alcoholism and drug abuse. *Gerontologist, 17*(2): 168-174, 1977.

Schuckit, M.A., and Miller, P.L.: Alcoholism in elderly men: A survey of a general medical ward. *Ann. N.Y. Acad Sci, 273*:558-571, 1975.

Shore, H.: Designing a sensory training program for understanding sensory losses in aging. *Gerontologist, 16*(2), 1976.

Simon, A., Epstein, L., and Reynolds, L.: Alcoholism in the geriatric mentally ill. *Geriatrics, 23*:125-131, 1968.

Smith, W. Lynn, and Kinsbourne, Marcel (Eds.): *Aging and Dementia.* New York: Spectrum Publications, 1977.

Solomon, R.L., and Wynne, L.C.: Traumatic avoidance learning: The principles of anxiety conservation and partial irreversibility. *Psychological Review, 61*:353-395, 1954.

Sternlicht, D.: *Medicine, Drugs and the Elderly.* Fort Lauderdale, Florida: Health Communications, Inc., 1980.

Sunby, R.: *Alcoholism and Mortality.* Oslo: Universitets for laget, 1967.

Swift, H.A., and Williams, T.: *Recovery for the Whole Family.* Center City, Minnesota: Hazelden Foundation, 1975.

Tashiro, M., and Lipscomb, W.R.: Mortality experience of alcoholics. *Quart J Stud Alc, 24*:203–212, 1963.

Tiebout, H.M.: The ego factors in surrender in alcoholism. *Quarterly J Stud Alc, 15*:610–621, 1954.

Tiebout, H.M.: *The Act of Surrender in the Therapeutic Process*. New York: The National Council on Alcoholism, Inc., 1939.

Treas, J.: Family support systems for the aged. *Gerontologist, 17*:486–491, 1977.

"Twelve Steps and the Older Member." Older Member Press, of Alcoholics Anonymous Connecticut, (1964) U. S. Department of Health, Education and Welfare. "Alcohol: Some Questions and Answers." Rockville Maryland: U.S. Government Printing Office, 1971.

U. S. Department of Health and Human Resources: *Here's to Your Health: Alcohol Facts for Women*. Rockville, Maryland: U.S. Government Printing Office, 1981.

U. S. Department of Health, Education, and Welfare: *Second Special Report to the U. S. Congress on Alcohol and Health from the Secretary of Health, Education & Welfare* (DHEW Publ. No. ADM 75–212). Washington, D.C.: U.S. Government Printing Office, 1974.

U. S. Department of Health, Education and Welfare: *First Special Report to the U. S. Congress on Alcohol and Health from the Secretary of Health, Education and Welfare* (DHEW Publ. No. ADM 74–68). Washington, D.C.: U.S. Government Printing Office, 1971.

U. S. Department of Health and Human Services: *The Dementias: Hope through Research* (NIH No. 81–2252). Bethesda, MD.: U.S. Government Printing Office, 1981.

U. S. Department of Health and Human Services: *Alzheimer's Disease: Questions and Answers* (NIH Publication No. 80–1646). Bethesda, MD.: U.S. Government Printing Office, 1980.

U. S. Department of Health and Human Services: *Alzheimer's Disease: A Scientific Guide for Health Practitioners* (NIH Publication No. 81–2251). Rockville, MD.: U.S. Government Printing Office, 1980.

U. S. Department of HEW: *Fact Sheet: Senile Dementia (Alzheimer's Disease)* (No. ADM 80–929). Rockville, MD.: U.S. Government Printing Office, 1980.

Wagman, R.I. (Ed.): *The New Complete Medical and Health Encylopedia*. Chicago: Ferguson Publishing Co., 1974, vol. 4.

Wagman, R.I. (Ed.): *The New Complete Medical and Health Encyclopedic*. Chicago: Ferguson Publishing Co., 1974, vol. 3.

Walker, B., and Kelly, P.: *The Elderly: A Guide for Counselors*. Center City, Minnesota: Hazelden Foundation 1981.

Waller, J.A.: Factors associated with alcohol and responsibility for highway crashes. *Quar J Stud Alc, 33*:160–170, 1972.

Waller, J.A.: Traffic accidents and violations. *Quart J Stud Alc, 39*:120–128, 1978.

Weg, R.B.: Changing physiology of aging: Normal and pathological. In Woodruff, D.S., and Berren, J.E.: *Aging: Scientific Perspectives and Social Issues.* New York: Van Nostrand Co., 1975.

Wegner, M.: *Diagnosis: Alcoholic.* Center City, Minnesota: Hazelden Foundation, 1981.

Wegscheider, D., and Wegscheider, S.: *Family Illness: Chemical Dependency.* Crystal, Minnesota: Nurturing Networks, 1978.

Wegscheider, S.: *The Family Trap . . . No One Escapes From a Chemically Dependent Family.* Crystal, Minnesota: Nurturing Networks, 1979.

Wegscheider, S., and Wegscheider, D.: *If Only My Family Understood Me.* Minneapolis: CompCare Publications, 1979.

Wegscheider, S.: *Another Chance: Hope and Help for Alcoholic Families.* Palo Alto, CA: Science and Behavior, 1981.

Weinberg, J.R.: *Sex and Recovery.* Center City, Minnesota: Recovery Press, 1977.

Weinberg, J.R.: *Helping the Client with Alcohol-Related Problems.* Minneapolis: CompCare Publications, 1973.

Zarit, S.H.: *Aging and Mental Disorders.* New York: Free Press, 1980.

Zink, M.: *Ways to Live More Comfortably with Your Alcoholic.* Minneapolis: CompCare Publications, 1977.

Zylman, R.: Single cause explanation. *Quart J Stud Alc., 39*:212-219, 1978.

INDEX